McGraw-Hill Education

5TEAS
Practice
Tests

McGraw-Hill Education

5 TEAS Practice Tests

Third Edition

Kathy A. Zahler
Wendy Hanks

New York Chicago San Francisco Athens London Madrid
Mexico City Milan New Delhi Singapore Sydney Toronto

1 2 3 4 5 6 7 8 9   LHS   22 21 20 19 18 17

ISBN   978-1-259-86344-8
MHID   1-259-86344-1

e-ISBN 978-1-259-86345-5
e-MHID   1-259-86345-X

McGraw-Hill Education products are available at special quantity discounts for use as premiums and sales promotions, or for use in corporate training programs. To contact a representative, please visit the Contact Us pages at www.mhprofessional.com.

TEAS is a trademark of Assessment Technologies Institute™ LLC, which was not involved in the production of, and does not endorse, this product.

For Paul and Olivia

Contents

SECTION I

INTRODUCTION TO THE TEAS

ALL ABOUT THE TEAS

This book contains five practice tests for the TEAS® (Test of Essential Academic Skills). The TEAS replaced the TEAS V and is the version most likely to be required by nursing schools today. Taking these practice tests will give you a good idea of what you'll encounter when you take the real exam. As you complete the tests, you'll become familiar with the directions, structure, and content that you're likely to see when you take the real exam.

TEAS Versus Other Nursing School Exams

WHO TAKES THE TEAS EXAM?

The TEAS exam is used for admission to certain nursing schools. It is administered by the Assessment Technologies Institute (ATI) of Leawood, Kansas. Different programs require different exams; for example, some schools expect applicants to take the Nurse Entrance Test (NET) or the National League for Nursing Pre-Admission Examination (NLN PAX-RN). Other schools give you a variety of entrance exams from which to choose. Still others require the TEAS exclusively.

HOW DO I KNOW WHETHER I SHOULD TAKE THE TEAS EXAM?

To know whether the school or schools of your choice require the TEAS, visit their websites or call their admissions offices. Before you begin to study, make sure that you are studying for the correct test.

Planning to Take the TEAS

WHEN IS THE TEAS GIVEN, AND HOW DO I REGISTER FOR IT?

The test is given at testing sites around the country, often at nursing schools or community colleges. The dates of the test depend on the application dates for the nursing school where you take the test. Some sites offer only online testing, others offer only paper-and-pencil versions of the test, and some offer both.

Before you take the test, you must log onto the ATI website and set up an account—www.atitesting.com. Remember the username and password you use for your account—you will need them when you log in for the electronic version of the test. Test sites are listed on the website. You will also need to register at the testing site and pay a fee as designated by that site.

WHEN SHOULD I TAKE THE TEAS?

You have the option of designating recipients of your transcript when you take the test. It may take up to 48 hours for scores to be sent out. Check with your chosen nursing programs to find out when they need score transcripts. Then work backward from that date to determine when you should take the test.

If you take the test at the nursing school that you hope to attend, the date of the test will be designed to mesh with that school's application dates.

WHAT DO I NEED ON THE DAY OF THE TEST?

If you are taking a pencil-and-paper version of the test, you will need several sharpened number 2 pencils with erasers that work well and erase thoroughly. If you are taking the TEAS online, you will need your ATI account username and password. For either form of the test, you must present one form of government-issued identification. Passports, driver's licenses, or green cards are fine; credit card photos or student IDs are not.

You may not bring in any resources such as calculators or reference books. A basic calculator will be given to you by the testing center. This is the only calculator that you may use. You may not carry a cell phone, pager, or other electronic device. You may not bring food or beverages into the testing site.

Scoring the TEAS

HOW IS THE TEAS SCORED?

You will receive a printed transcript, which will include a variety of numbers. In the top right corner is your *adjusted composite score*, which is the number of correct answers divided by the total number of questions, adjusted for the difficulty level of the test you took. Below that number is the *national mean*, which is the average of the adjusted composite scores for all people who took this particular version of the test. Below that is the *program mean*, which is the average of the adjusted composite scores for all people who took this particular version of the test and are in a program similar to yours. Below that are the *national percentile rank* and the *program percentile rank*. These figures show how you rate compared to other people who took the test.

A table below these headings shows the breakdown of skills—how you performed in the various subcategories within the tested areas of reading, mathematics, science, and English and language usage. Some schools look specifically at these breakdowns; others may only be interested in your adjusted composite score.

WHEN WILL I RECEIVE MY SCORE?

At the end of your electronic test, you will receive a printed score report. The facility where you took your test will be able to access that score online. If you take a pencil-and-paper version of the test, you should receive your scores within 48 hours.

HOW DO I SUBMIT MY SCORE TO NURSING PROGRAMS?

Your testing fee automatically includes the submission of scores to the facility where you took the test. If you want your transcript sent to other schools as well, it will cost you $27 per additional school. You can order transcripts, which are sent immediately via e-mail, by logging onto the ATI website at www.atitesting.com/ati_store/.

IS MY SCORE GOOD ENOUGH?

That depends on the program to which you are applying. Some nursing schools have specific cutoff points for each category—reading, mathematics, science, and English and language usage. Others accept entrants who have achieved a score equal to or better than the national average for that day's test. Still others give greatest weight to the science section of the test. Many nursing schools look at the adjusted composite score, which is made up of the average score of all four sections. ATI will not interpret your scores; you must contact the nursing program of your choice to do that for you.

Some nursing programs allow you to take the TEAS three times or more if your first scores are unacceptable. Again, the rules vary from program to program.

PARTS OF THE TEST

The TEAS is divided into four content areas: reading, mathematics, science, and English and language usage. This chart shows the number of items and the time allotted for each section.

Content Area	Number of Items	Time Allotted
Reading	53	64 minutes
Mathematics	36	54 minutes
Science	53	63 minutes
English and Language Usage	28	28 minutes
TOTAL	170	209 minutes

The numbers given are for the ATI TEAS only. Earlier versions of the test have different numbers of items.

> **Format Tip**
>
> Twenty TEAS questions are experimental, unscored items. As you take the test, you will not know which items those are. The number of scored items on the TEAS is 150.

Reading

Reading items test paragraph and passage comprehension and informational source comprehension. You may be asked to read a multiparagraph passage and answer a variety of questions about it. You should also expect to be asked to read and interpret labels, directions, graphs, charts, measuring tools, and maps.

Some of the most common reading skills tested on the TEAS are the following:

- Identifying the author's purpose or intent
- Distinguishing fact from opinion
- Identifying genre
- Distinguishing among topic, main idea, theme, and supporting details
- Identifying topic and summary sentences
- Drawing conclusions and making inferences
- Making logical predictions
- Evaluating an argument
- Identifying primary sources
- Sequencing events
- Synthesizing information from multiple sources
- Identifying text features or structure
- Defining vocabulary

Format Tip

All questions on the TEAS are multiple-choice. All questions have four possible answer choices labeled A, B, C, and D.

Here are two examples of TEAS reading questions.

Dear Clients:

We wish to apologize for any inconvenience to you resulting from our server's being down on Monday, May 18. High winds in the area caused a power outage, and it took longer than expected to get things up and running again. Rest assured that we are back on track and that no materials were lost. Again, we are sorry for the delay.

Sincerely,

Robert Dullea

1. Which of the following is the author's main purpose in writing this passage?

   A) To assess his clients' level of concern
   B) To apologize and reassure his clients
   C) To explain how wind may affect data
   D) To obtain new clients for his business

Explanatory Answer: This question tests your understanding of the author's purpose or intent. This author's intent appears in his opening sentence. He does not ask for a response from the client; if he had, choice A might make sense. Although he blames the problem on wind, he does not go into an explanation of how it affected data (choice C). He is clearly writing to existing clients, not to potential ones (choice D). The best answer is choice B.

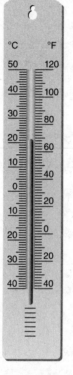

2. What measurement is represented on the thermometer above?

A) 21°C
B) 21°F
C) 60°C
D) 60°F

Explanatory Answer: This question tests your ability to read a measuring tool. The left-hand scale shows degrees Celsius; the right-hand scale shows degrees Fahrenheit. The colored column reaches to about 21 degrees on the left-hand scale and around 70 degrees on the right-hand scale. The best answer is choice A.

Mathematics

Mathematics items test your knowledge of numbers and operations, measurement, data interpretation, and algebraic applications. Common skills tested include the following:

• Adding, subtracting, multiplying, and dividing fractions
• Converting among fractions, decimals, and percents

- Comparing numbers
- Estimating answers
- Determining costs
- Calculating interest or tips
- Solving problems involving ratios and proportions
- Converting measurements
- Interpreting graphs and charts
- Solving algebraic expressions

Format Tip

Sometimes, two or more questions will refer to a single graph, chart, or passage.

Here are two examples of TEAS mathematics questions.

1. Subtract and simplify $2\dfrac{11}{12} - \dfrac{3}{16}$.

A) $1\dfrac{7}{8}$

B) $2\dfrac{1}{8}$

C) $2\dfrac{5}{6}$

D) $2\dfrac{35}{48}$

Explanatory Answer: To add or subtract fractions, first find the lowest common denominator and convert each fraction to an equivalent fraction with that denominator. Here, the lowest common denominator is 48.

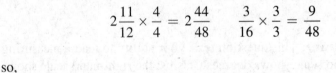

$$2\dfrac{11}{12} \times \dfrac{4}{4} = 2\dfrac{44}{48} \qquad \dfrac{3}{16} \times \dfrac{3}{3} = \dfrac{9}{48}$$

so,

$$2\dfrac{44}{48} - \dfrac{9}{48} = 2\dfrac{35}{48}$$

That fraction cannot be reduced further, so the best answer is choice D.

2. How many kilograms are there in 98 grams?

A) 0.0098 kilograms
B) 0.098 kilograms
C) 0.98 kilograms
D) 9.8 kilograms

Explanatory Answer: This question tests your ability to convert measurements. Think: Since 1,000 grams = 1 kilogram, 9,000 grams = 9 kilograms. Therefore, 900 grams = 0.9 kilograms, and 90 grams = 0.09 kilograms. Knowing that, you can see that 98 grams = 0.098 kilograms. The correct answer is choice B.

Science

The science section mainly tests four categories: science of the human body, life science, physical science, and scientific reasoning. Questions might focus on any of the following skills, among others:

- Identifying organs, systems, and functions
- Understanding DNA and RNA
- Recognizing basic nutritional principles
- Identifying parts of a cell
- Identifying properties of macromolecules
- Contrasting respiration and photosynthesis
- Contrasting meiosis and mitosis
- Using taxonomy
- Determining phenotypes and genotypes
- Interpreting a Punnett square
- Using the periodic table of elements
- Identifying properties of atoms
- Recognizing properties of matter
- Interpreting pH scale values
- Understanding chemical bonds
- Identifying chemical reactions
- Identifying the parts of an experiment
- Interpreting a scientific argument
- Suggesting future experiments
- Identifying appropriate scientific tools

Here are two examples of TEAS science questions.

1. How does the muscular system work with the endocrine system?

   A) The endocrine system coordinates general muscle activity.
   B) The muscular system generates chemicals for the endocrine system.
   C) Hormones from the endocrine system determine muscle strength.
   D) The endocrine system provides protection for certain muscles.

Explanatory Answer: This human body question asks you to identify how organ systems work together. The endocrine system does not coordinate muscle activity, the nervous system does; so choice A is wrong. Choices B and D reverse the actions of the two systems. Hormones are responsible for growth and muscle strength, making choice C the correct answer.

2. Why does the pressure of gas in a closed, rigid container increase when the temperature of the gas increases?

A) The density of the gas increases.
B) The container expands as it warms.
C) The heated gas molecules bond together and increase in mass.
D) The rate of collisions of gas molecules with the surface increases.

Explanatory Answer: This question tests your understanding of some basic properties of matter. As gas is heated, its molecules have more energy and collide with more force, increasing the pressure in a sealed container. Although the container expands slightly when heated (choice B), this does not increase the pressure and might in fact slightly decrease it. The correct answer is choice D.

Format Tip

Occasional ATI TEAS questions will require the interpretation of diagrams and illustrations.

English and Language Usage

The last section of the TEAS deals with grammar, word meaning, spelling, punctuation, and sentence structure. Here are some of the subskills that you might see on the test:

- Identifying parts of speech
- Identifying pronoun antecedents
- Making subjects and verbs agree
- Using verb tenses correctly
- Defining difficult vocabulary
- Distinguishing among multiple meanings
- Using the correct homophone
- Spelling irregular plurals
- Spelling compound or hyphenated words
- Spelling frequently misspelled words
- Identifying correctly punctuated sentences
- Capitalizing names, titles, and addresses correctly
- Distinguishing among simple, compound, and complex sentences
- Clarifying sentence structure
- Differentiating first- from third-person point of view
- Changing passive to active voice
- Distinguishing formal from informal language
- Understanding parts of the writing process
- Structuring paragraphs
- Using word parts to define words

Here are two examples of TEAS English and language usage questions.

1. Which of the following nouns is written in the correct plural form?

A) crises
B) bacterias
C) sheeps
D) rooves

Explanatory Answer: This spelling question asks you to identify the correct irregular plural. The plural of *bacterium* is *bacteria* (choice B), the plural of *sheep* is *sheep* (choice C), and the plural of *roof* is *roofs* (choice D). Because the plural of *crisis* is *crises*, the correct answer is choice A.

2. Which of the following is an example of a compound sentence?

A) Jasper especially loves playing with the marching band.
B) Jasper and his bandmates are heading to a competition.
C) Jasper plays the trombone, but he is taking sax lessons, too.
D) When the band performs, people in the bleachers dance.

Explanatory Answer: This question asks you to differentiate among types of sentences. Choice A is a simple sentence with one subject and one verb. Choice B has a compound subject, but it is not a compound sentence. Choice D is a complex sentence with one dependent and one independent clause. The answer is choice C; it consists of two independent clauses separated by a comma and a conjunction.

SECTION II

TIPS AND STRATEGIES FOR TEST-TAKERS

HOW TO USE THIS BOOK

Preparing for the TEAS ahead of time is worth the effort. This book will help you to do the following:

- Familiarize yourself with the test format.
- Recognize the skills tested on the TEAS.
- Practice your test-taking skills using sample TEASs.

Here is a practical study program that will help you to make the best use of this book. The amount of study and review you do between tests will depend on those weaknesses you discover as you assess your responses and compare them to the explanatory answers that follow each test.

Step 1. Think about Your Weaknesses

If it has been a long time since you took biology or thought about parts of speech or algebraic equations, you might want to brush up on those long-lost skills. Section I of this book (pages 5–11) lists the major skills that are covered on the TEAS. Build some review time into your test-prep schedule. Pull out your old textbooks, go to the library, or do some online review.

Step 2. Take the Practice Tests

There are five practice tests, and each one is designed to take 209 minutes (3 hours and 29 minutes), just as the real TEAS does. Do not take more than one practice test a day. As you take each test, try to simulate actual test conditions. Sit in a quiet room, time yourself, and work through as much of the test as time allows. If you wish, take a break after each section of the test. When you are done, check your answers against the explanatory answers that follow the test you took. Use the explanatory answers to figure out what you did right and where you went wrong.

In *McGraw-Hill Education: 5 TEAS Practice Tests*, practice tests 1, 3, and 5 are designed to be parallel, as are practice tests 2 and 4. This means that *in most cases*, similarly numbered questions on tests 1, 3, and 5 will measure the same sort of skill, as will similarly numbered questions on tests 2 and 4. This fact will help you determine where your problem areas are. For example, if you consistently miss question number 34 in the mathematics section of practice tests 1, 3, and 5, you can assume that you need to study up on the concept of ratios.

If you are sure that you will end up taking an online version of the test, and you would like to know what that experience is like, you may visit www.atitesting.com and pay to take an online practice test. At the end of the test, you will receive a score report and a list of skills and concepts to review.

Step 3. Review and Improve

Each time you take a practice test, review the explanatory answers. Give yourself a break of a few days. Then take another practice test and see whether you do better. Look for patterns as you continue to take practice tests. Do you miss the same kinds of questions on each practice test you take? Make a list of skills to review, and do some serious studying before you take the final two practice tests. If you have kept track of your weaknesses and studied those skills in depth, you should see a noticeable improvement in your score.

STRATEGIES FOR TOP SCORES

As with any test, you can use certain strategies to improve your TEAS score. You already know whether you are better at math or at science, or whether your English language skills are adequate. Now it's important to learn about the test itself and what to expect on test day.

Study Strategies

- **Get to know the format of the exam.** The practice tests in this book are designed to be similar to what you will see on the TEAS.
- **Get to know the test directions.** The TEAS is not different from other multiple-choice tests you have taken over the years. There are always four choices, and most questions are stand-alone. When more than one question refers to a single passage or diagram, that fact is explained in a direction line.
- **Get to know what topics are covered.** Section I (pages 5–11) lists the major skills that are covered on the TEAS.
- **Test and review.** If possible, give yourself time to take each of the practice tests in this book. These are long tests, so you will need to map out big chunks of time with breaks in between. Do not plan to take more than one test in a day. Review the answers, look for patterns, and review those skills that consistently cause problems for you.

Test-Taking Strategies

- **Answer all the questions, but go back if you have time.** Your time is limited on each section of the test—in particular, TEAS test-takers often complain that they have too little time for the math section—so try to answer each question as you go. However, keep track on scratch paper of those questions that give you trouble. If you have time at the end of the section, go back and readdress those questions, and change your answers if you wish. Even the online version of the test allows you to go back and change answers within a given section. (You will not be able to go back once you've completed a section and moved to a new section, however.)

- **Use the process of elimination.** Even if you feel completely stumped, you will probably be able to eliminate one or more choices simply by using common sense. That improves your odds of getting the right answer.
- **When in doubt, guess.** On the TEAS, every question has the same value, and there are no points taken off for guessing. Use the process of elimination, but if you're baffled, go ahead and guess. You have a 25 percent chance of getting the answer right. If you leave the answer blank, your chance drops to 0.
- **Beware of answer choices that look reasonable but are not correct.** Because the choices on the TEAS are multiple-choice, the test-makers have many chances to mislead you with tricky distractors (wrong answers). Focus, use scratch paper to solve problems, and use the process of elimination to help narrow your choices.

Tips for Test Day

- **Get a good night's sleep.** You need energy to face a test that is more than 3 hours long, and you won't have energy if you're exhausted from worry or from excessive, last-minute review. If you have taken all your practice tests, reviewed those skills that troubled you, and improved your scores on your final tests, you have done what you need to do to succeed. Arriving at the test site well rested and alert will improve your chances dramatically.
- **Be careful as you indicate your answers.** If you take the pencil-and-paper TEAS, your answer sheet will be machine-scored, so mark it carefully. Fill in answer ovals completely, erase thoroughly if necessary, and do not make any stray marks anywhere on the sheet. Be sure that the answer space you are marking matches the number of the question you are answering. If you skip a question, skip the corresponding space on the answer sheet. Use your finger to hold your place if it helps. If you are taking the test on computer, the TEAS allows you to move back and forth freely. Just take care not to skip any questions.
- **Watch the time.** Wear a watch and check yourself from time to time. If you have timed yourself on the practice tests, you should be pretty good at estimating the time you have left as you progress through the TEAS. The online version of the TEAS has a toolbar that keeps track of your time for each section of the test.
- **Use any extra time to go back and fix answers.** If you are unsure of some answers, take time at the end of the section to go back and change them if necessary. Remember, even if you need to guess, you're better off answering a question than skipping it entirely.

TEAS TRAINING SCHEDULE

Are you ready to get started? Use this sample schedule to plan your attack.

MY TEAS TEST-PREP SCHEDULE

Test Center: _____

Date: _____ **Time:** _____

4 Weeks Before	Register for the test via www.atitesting.com Take Practice Test 1	Number of correct answers divided by 170 questions: Problem Areas:
3 Weeks Before	Take Practice Test 2 Take Practice Test 3 Review	Number of correct answers divided by 170 questions: Number of correct answers divided by 170 questions: Problem Areas: Test 3 compared to Test 1:
2 Weeks Before	Take Practice Test 4 Take Practice Test 5 Review	Number of correct answers divided by 170 questions: Number of correct answers divided by 170 questions: Problem Areas: Test 4 compared to Test 2: Test 5 compared to Test 3:
1 Week Before	Consider taking an online practice test at www. atitesting.com Review	Score: Skills & concepts to review:

SECTION III

5 TEAS PRACTICE TESTS

TEAS PRACTICE TEST 1

TEAS Practice Test 1: Answer Sheet

READING

1 Ⓐ Ⓑ Ⓒ Ⓓ	19 Ⓐ Ⓑ Ⓒ Ⓓ	37 Ⓐ Ⓑ Ⓒ Ⓓ
2 Ⓐ Ⓑ Ⓒ Ⓓ	20 Ⓐ Ⓑ Ⓒ Ⓓ	38 Ⓐ Ⓑ Ⓒ Ⓓ
3 Ⓐ Ⓑ Ⓒ Ⓓ	21 Ⓐ Ⓑ Ⓒ Ⓓ	39 Ⓐ Ⓑ Ⓒ Ⓓ
4 Ⓐ Ⓑ Ⓒ Ⓓ	22 Ⓐ Ⓑ Ⓒ Ⓓ	40 Ⓐ Ⓑ Ⓒ Ⓓ
5 Ⓐ Ⓑ Ⓒ Ⓓ	23 Ⓐ Ⓑ Ⓒ Ⓓ	41 Ⓐ Ⓑ Ⓒ Ⓓ
6 Ⓐ Ⓑ Ⓒ Ⓓ	24 Ⓐ Ⓑ Ⓒ Ⓓ	42 Ⓐ Ⓑ Ⓒ Ⓓ
7 Ⓐ Ⓑ Ⓒ Ⓓ	25 Ⓐ Ⓑ Ⓒ Ⓓ	43 Ⓐ Ⓑ Ⓒ Ⓓ
8 Ⓐ Ⓑ Ⓒ Ⓓ	26 Ⓐ Ⓑ Ⓒ Ⓓ	44 Ⓐ Ⓑ Ⓒ Ⓓ
9 Ⓐ Ⓑ Ⓒ Ⓓ	27 Ⓐ Ⓑ Ⓒ Ⓓ	45 Ⓐ Ⓑ Ⓒ Ⓓ
10 Ⓐ Ⓑ Ⓒ Ⓓ	28 Ⓐ Ⓑ Ⓒ Ⓓ	46 Ⓐ Ⓑ Ⓒ Ⓓ
11 Ⓐ Ⓑ Ⓒ Ⓓ	29 Ⓐ Ⓑ Ⓒ Ⓓ	47 Ⓐ Ⓑ Ⓒ Ⓓ
12 Ⓐ Ⓑ Ⓒ Ⓓ	30 Ⓐ Ⓑ Ⓒ Ⓓ	48 Ⓐ Ⓑ Ⓒ Ⓓ
13 Ⓐ Ⓑ Ⓒ Ⓓ	31 Ⓐ Ⓑ Ⓒ Ⓓ	49 Ⓐ Ⓑ Ⓒ Ⓓ
14 Ⓐ Ⓑ Ⓒ Ⓓ	32 Ⓐ Ⓑ Ⓒ Ⓓ	50 Ⓐ Ⓑ Ⓒ Ⓓ
15 Ⓐ Ⓑ Ⓒ Ⓓ	33 Ⓐ Ⓑ Ⓒ Ⓓ	51 Ⓐ Ⓑ Ⓒ Ⓓ
16 Ⓐ Ⓑ Ⓒ Ⓓ	34 Ⓐ Ⓑ Ⓒ Ⓓ	52 Ⓐ Ⓑ Ⓒ Ⓓ
17 Ⓐ Ⓑ Ⓒ Ⓓ	35 Ⓐ Ⓑ Ⓒ Ⓓ	53 Ⓐ Ⓑ Ⓒ Ⓓ
18 Ⓐ Ⓑ Ⓒ Ⓓ	36 Ⓐ Ⓑ Ⓒ Ⓓ	

MATHEMATICS

1 Ⓐ Ⓑ Ⓒ Ⓓ	13 Ⓐ Ⓑ Ⓒ Ⓓ	25 Ⓐ Ⓑ Ⓒ Ⓓ
2 Ⓐ Ⓑ Ⓒ Ⓓ	14 Ⓐ Ⓑ Ⓒ Ⓓ	26 Ⓐ Ⓑ Ⓒ Ⓓ
3 Ⓐ Ⓑ Ⓒ Ⓓ	15 Ⓐ Ⓑ Ⓒ Ⓓ	27 Ⓐ Ⓑ Ⓒ Ⓓ
4 Ⓐ Ⓑ Ⓒ Ⓓ	16 Ⓐ Ⓑ Ⓒ Ⓓ	28 Ⓐ Ⓑ Ⓒ Ⓓ
5 Ⓐ Ⓑ Ⓒ Ⓓ	17 Ⓐ Ⓑ Ⓒ Ⓓ	29 Ⓐ Ⓑ Ⓒ Ⓓ
6 Ⓐ Ⓑ Ⓒ Ⓓ	18 Ⓐ Ⓑ Ⓒ Ⓓ	30 Ⓐ Ⓑ Ⓒ Ⓓ
7 Ⓐ Ⓑ Ⓒ Ⓓ	19 Ⓐ Ⓑ Ⓒ Ⓓ	31 Ⓐ Ⓑ Ⓒ Ⓓ
8 Ⓐ Ⓑ Ⓒ Ⓓ	20 Ⓐ Ⓑ Ⓒ Ⓓ	32 Ⓐ Ⓑ Ⓒ Ⓓ
9 Ⓐ Ⓑ Ⓒ Ⓓ	21 Ⓐ Ⓑ Ⓒ Ⓓ	33 Ⓐ Ⓑ Ⓒ Ⓓ
10 Ⓐ Ⓑ Ⓒ Ⓓ	22 Ⓐ Ⓑ Ⓒ Ⓓ	34 Ⓐ Ⓑ Ⓒ Ⓓ
11 Ⓐ Ⓑ Ⓒ Ⓓ	23 Ⓐ Ⓑ Ⓒ Ⓓ	35 Ⓐ Ⓑ Ⓒ Ⓓ
12 Ⓐ Ⓑ Ⓒ Ⓓ	24 Ⓐ Ⓑ Ⓒ Ⓓ	36 Ⓐ Ⓑ Ⓒ Ⓓ

SCIENCE

1. (A) (B) (C) (D)
2. (A) (B) (C) (D)
3. (A) (B) (C) (D)
4. (A) (B) (C) (D)
5. (A) (B) (C) (D)
6. (A) (B) (C) (D)
7. (A) (B) (C) (D)
8. (A) (B) (C) (D)
9. (A) (B) (C) (D)
10. (A) (B) (C) (D)
11. (A) (B) (C) (D)
12. (A) (B) (C) (D)
13. (A) (B) (C) (D)
14. (A) (B) (C) (D)
15. (A) (B) (C) (D)
16. (A) (B) (C) (D)
17. (A) (B) (C) (D)
18. (A) (B) (C) (D)

19. (A) (B) (C) (D)
20. (A) (B) (C) (D)
21. (A) (B) (C) (D)
22. (A) (B) (C) (D)
23. (A) (B) (C) (D)
24. (A) (B) (C) (D)
25. (A) (B) (C) (D)
26. (A) (B) (C) (D)
27. (A) (B) (C) (D)
28. (A) (B) (C) (D)
29. (A) (B) (C) (D)
30. (A) (B) (C) (D)
31. (A) (B) (C) (D)
32. (A) (B) (C) (D)
33. (A) (B) (C) (D)
34. (A) (B) (C) (D)
35. (A) (B) (C) (D)
36. (A) (B) (C) (D)

37. (A) (B) (C) (D)
38. (A) (B) (C) (D)
39. (A) (B) (C) (D)
40. (A) (B) (C) (D)
41. (A) (B) (C) (D)
42. (A) (B) (C) (D)
43. (A) (B) (C) (D)
44. (A) (B) (C) (D)
45. (A) (B) (C) (D)
46. (A) (B) (C) (D)
47. (A) (B) (C) (D)
48. (A) (B) (C) (D)
49. (A) (B) (C) (D)
50. (A) (B) (C) (D)
51. (A) (B) (C) (D)
52. (A) (B) (C) (D)
53. (A) (B) (C) (D)

ENGLISH AND LANGUAGE USAGE

1. (A) (B) (C) (D)
2. (A) (B) (C) (D)
3. (A) (B) (C) (D)
4. (A) (B) (C) (D)
5. (A) (B) (C) (D)
6. (A) (B) (C) (D)
7. (A) (B) (C) (D)
8. (A) (B) (C) (D)
9. (A) (B) (C) (D)
10. (A) (B) (C) (D)

11. (A) (B) (C) (D)
12. (A) (B) (C) (D)
13. (A) (B) (C) (D)
14. (A) (B) (C) (D)
15. (A) (B) (C) (D)
16. (A) (B) (C) (D)
17. (A) (B) (C) (D)
18. (A) (B) (C) (D)
19. (A) (B) (C) (D)
20. (A) (B) (C) (D)

21. (A) (B) (C) (D)
22. (A) (B) (C) (D)
23. (A) (B) (C) (D)
24. (A) (B) (C) (D)
25. (A) (B) (C) (D)
26. (A) (B) (C) (D)
27. (A) (B) (C) (D)
28. (A) (B) (C) (D)

Part I. Reading

53 items (47 scored), 64 minutes

Jason Trains for the Triathlon

In spring, Jason decided to train for the triathlon. Several of his friends had tried it the autumn before, and they all vouched for its being not only possible, but also loads of fun.

He began by signing up with the local Triathlon Club. The people there offered good advice, companionship, and a premade series of running and biking maps. He started slowly, as recommended by his new friends. By summer, he was biking 20 miles daily and running at least 5 miles.

It was the swimming that confounded him. He had never been a very strong swimmer, and he hated training at the local pool. There were never enough free lanes, and small children splashed him and messed up his timing.

"You can find someone else to do the swimming part," a friend advised him. "You should concentrate on the two things you do well."

Jason wasn't ready to give up. As the weather warmed up, he went regularly to the lake and swam back and forth, back and forth. His lungs felt like bursting, and his legs shook when he emerged, but he could feel himself getting stronger and more secure in the water.

As a beginner, he would do the Sprint course this year. That meant swimming 750 meters, then biking 20 kilometers, and finally running 5 kilometers. The swimming came first. If he failed to make it through that part, the easier pieces would never happen at all.

The day arrived, and Jason received his number and prepared with hundreds of others to enter the water. The age range was remarkable; swimmers ranged from teenagers to octogenarians. In a flash, Jason was in the water with the others, avoiding kicking legs and splashing arms. Within a moment or two, he knew he could do it. He found his rhythm, pulled steadily, and ignored the noise and spray. The months of training had paid off for Jason. He was on his way to completing his first triathlon!

The next seven questions are based on this passage.

1. Does the title of the passage reflect the passage's theme, topic, main idea, or supporting details?

   A) Theme
   B) Topic
   C) Main idea
   D) Supporting details

GO ON TO THE NEXT PAGE

2. Why did the author probably write this passage?

    A) To tell an inspiring story
    B) To persuade reluctant athletes
    C) To give step-by-step directions
    D) To reflect on a personal accomplishment

3. What can you conclude about the Triathlon Club members from the second paragraph of the passage?

    A) They are extremely competitive.
    B) They are welcoming and helpful.
    C) They are older than Jason.
    D) They win most of the races they enter.

4. Which sentence from the passage expresses an opinion?

    A) "You should concentrate on the two things you do well."
    B) "You can find someone else to do the swimming part."
    C) By summer, he was biking 20 miles daily and running at least 5 miles.
    D) He found his rhythm, pulled steadily, and ignored the noise and spray.

5. Which of the following inferences may logically be drawn from the sixth paragraph of the passage?

    A) Advanced triathletes compete in a longer course.
    B) Beginning triathletes perform two out of three tasks.
    C) All triathletes must swim a maximum of 750 meters.
    D) Triathletes must swim and run before they bicycle.

6. Which aspect of this passage does *not* mark it as narrative writing?

    A) Made-up character
    B) Sequential order of events
    C) Facts about a sport
    D) Use of dialogue

7. Which of the following might serve as a summary statement for the passage?

    A) It was the swimming that confounded him.
    B) As a beginner, he would do the Sprint course this year.
    C) The months of training had paid off for Jason.
    D) Within a moment or two, he knew he could do it.

GO ON TO THE NEXT PAGE

Dear Editor:

It has come to my attention that our county's planning commission is wedded to the concept of nodal development in our rural towns. This concept is problematic for several reasons.

To succeed, nodes must have a critical mass of inhabitants. Studies suggest that 2,500 is the smallest possible group required to support retail businesses within a node. Our rural nodes would have far fewer residents—at most, 1,500.

Nodes do best when they are part of existing suburbs and exurbs. Those are the places where citizens want the option of walking to stores and schools while still having access to larger structures in the cities. Rural communities, on the other hand, rely on outside access to their businesses in order to survive.

I strongly encourage our planning commission to look toward our existing hamlets and villages as the centers of life in our rural towns. Imposing an urban structure on rural towns can only lead to disaster.

Sincerely,

Lawrence Simon

The next five questions are based on this passage.

8. Which of the following is a likely motive for the author?

   A) He wants a position on the county's planning commission.
   B) He wants the county to improve its urban centers.
   C) He wants the planning commission to choose a different path.
   D) He wants rural nodes to look more like those in the suburbs.

9. Which of the following inferences may logically be drawn from the letter?

   A) The author is a resident of a nodal development.
   B) The author and his readers live in a fairly rural area.
   C) The author moved from the city to enjoy a rural life.
   D) The author is either a trained architect or a city planner.

10. The passage is reflective of which of the following types of writing?

   A) Persuasive
   B) Narrative
   C) Expository
   D) Technical

GO ON TO THE NEXT PAGE

11. Which of the following reflects the author's point of view about nodal development?

    A) It works in some places but not in others.
    B) It is never an appropriate course of action.
    C) It is especially useful in smaller communities.
    D) It is a good way to merge rural and urban life.

12. The third paragraph is reflective of which of the following types of text structures?

    A) Cause-effect
    B) Comparison-contrast
    C) Sequence
    D) Problem-solution

Allergen patch tests are diagnostic tests applied to the surface of the skin. Physicians use patch tests to <u>establish</u> the specific causes of contact dermatitis. The patches are manufactured from natural substances or chemicals (such as nickel, rubber, and fragrance mixes) that are known to cause contact dermatitis.

The next two questions are based on this passage.

13. In this context, *establish* means

    A) launch.
    B) introduce.
    C) endorse.
    D) determine.

14. A diagnostic test is one that

    A) locates a cure.
    B) looks for a cause.
    C) examines the skin.
    D) is performed on doctors.

When it comes to philanthropists who hide their light under a bushel, it is possible that none is as shy as Marcella Thurston. Ms. Thurston's contributions to our local library, hospital, and city park have no equal, but she has not seen fit to append her name to any of her many projects. For that reason, and because of her continuing support for our cause, the County Fund has seen fit to honor her today.

The next two questions are based on this passage.

15. In the context of the passage, does the phrase "library, hospital, and city park" constitute a topic, a main idea, a theme, or supporting details?

    A) Topic
    B) Main idea
    C) Theme
    D) Supporting details

GO ON TO THE NEXT PAGE

16. What is the author's apparent purpose for writing this paragraph about Ms. Thurston?

A) To explain her motives
B) To praise and commend her
C) To provide her biography
D) To entertain the audience

Pricing Chart: Contact Lenses

Product	Description	Cost for One Month's Supply
EZ on the Eyes	daily lens; soft; clear	$74.95
Simply Bright	monthly lens; hard; tinted	$52.78
No-Scratch	monthly lens; scratch-resistant; hard; clear	$42.85
Liqui-Fill	daily lens; soft; clear	$78.40

The next two questions are based on this price listing.

17. Lucia wants a lens that changes her blue eyes to green. Which of the suggested lenses should she purchase?

A) EZ on the Eyes
B) Simply Bright
C) No-Scratch
D) Liqui-Fill

18. José prefers a lens that he can wear once and throw away. Which is the best and cheapest purchase for him?

A) EZ on the Eyes
B) Simply Bright
C) No-Scratch
D) Liqui-Fill

GO ON TO THE NEXT PAGE

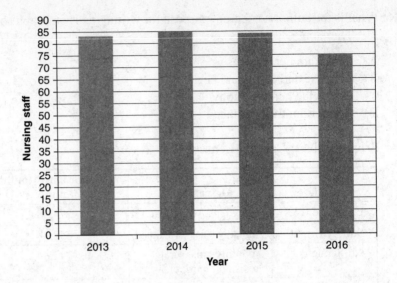

The next two questions are based on this graph.

19. In which years did the hospital have more than 80 nursing staff?

   A) Just 2014
   B) 2014 and 2015
   C) 2013 and 2014
   D) All but 2016

20. In which year did the hospital have the greatest number of nursing staff?

   A) 2013
   B) 2014
   C) 2015
   D) 2016

21. Read and follow the directions below.

   1. Imagine a deck of 52 cards.
   2. Remove all four queens.
   3. Add back the queen of hearts.
   4. Remove all four kings.
   5. Add back the king of spades.

   Which of the following tells the number of cards now in the deck?

   A) 46 cards
   B) 48 cards
   C) 50 cards
   D) 52 cards

GO ON TO THE NEXT PAGE

22. A student writing a report wants to make sure that she has replaced all trite and overused words with appropriate and interesting synonyms. Which of the following resources would be most appropriate for her to use?

A) *The Complete Rhyming Dictionary*
B) *English Composition and Grammar*
C) *Handy Dictionary of Poetical Quotations*
D) *Webster's New World Thesaurus*

23.

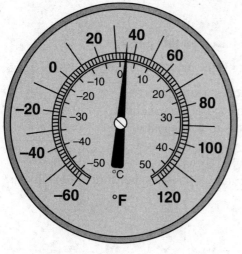

On the thermometer above, what is the current temperature in degrees Celsius?

A) 3°
B) 10°
C) 38°
D) 40°

GO ON TO THE NEXT PAGE

The following e-mail was sent by an employee to her boss.

Dan—

You asked us to provide the optimal schedule for completion of the Davis project. Assuming that the start date is firm, my team could easily complete our part of the project by March 31. I hope that this works with everyone else's projections.

Thanks,

Kate

The next two questions are based on this passage.

24. Which of the following is the main purpose of the e-mail?

    A) To respond to a request from the boss
    B) To comment on a proposal from a client
    C) To persuade the boss to do something
    D) To express a personal point of view

25. In the context of the e-mail, what does the word *optimal* mean?

    A) Most likely
    B) Least critical
    C) Most visual
    D) Best possible

26.   Verbals

        gerund, 93
        infinitive, 97–98
        participle, 88–89

    Verbs

        action, 16–17
        active voice, 166–167
        agreement with subject, 130–145

A student wants to learn more about the type of verbal known as the infinitive. Based on this excerpt from a grammar text's index, on which of the following pages should the student begin to look?

    A) 88
    B) 96
    C) 97
    D) 98

GO ON TO THE NEXT PAGE

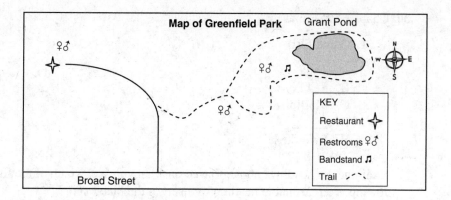

The next two questions are based on this map.

27. A family turns off Broad Street and heads to the restaurant in the park. In which two directions will they drive?

    A) West, then north
    B) North, then east
    C) West, then south
    D) North, then west

28. A hiker parks along the entry road and heads along the 2-mile trail around the pond. Approximately how far along will the hiker encounter the first restrooms?

    A) About $\frac{1}{4}$ mile in

    B) About $\frac{3}{4}$ mile in

    C) About 1 mile in

    D) About $1\frac{1}{2}$ miles in

29. Which of the following sentences indicates the start of a sequence of events?

    A) As soon as I heard his voice, I knew he was the right person.
    B) I asked the hotel clerk to connect me to Mr. Holder.
    C) Yesterday, I made an important overseas call.
    D) Before long, we were chatting like old friends.

GO ON TO THE NEXT PAGE

30. Chapter 5: Marine Fish

    1. Game Fish

        A. Tuna
        B. Sea Bass
        C. Marlin
        D. _____
        E. Swordfish

Examine the headings above. Based on what you see, which of the following is a reasonable heading to insert in the blank spot?

A) Aquariums
B) Mackerel
C) Corals
D) Anemones

31. Begin with the word *start*. Follow the directions to change the word.

    1. Remove the beginning letter and place it at the end.

    2. Change each *t* to *m*.

    3. Replace the first *m* with the letter *h*.

Which of the following is the new word?

A) arms
B) harm
C) tarts
D) harms

32. A student is interested in subletting her apartment for the summer while she takes an internship in another city. Which department of the newspaper should she contact?

A) Editorial
B) Classified
C) Local news
D) Business

33. Chapter 4: Languages of the Middle East

        A. Arabic
        B. Yoruba
        C. Persian
        D. Hebrew

GO ON TO THE NEXT PAGE

Analyze the headings on the preceding page. Which of the following headings is out of place?

A) Arabic
B) Yoruba
C) Persian
D) Hebrew

34. A historian is writing about Hurricane Katrina's effects on Louisiana. Which of the following would be a primary source she might use?

A) A magazine article about weather events in the 21st century
B) A guidebook to Louisiana and surrounding states
C) New Orleans hospital records from the time of the hurricane
D) Photographs of the hurricane from a recent photographic essay

35. A driver wishes to find the quickest route from Des Moines to Dubuque. Which of the following is the most appropriate source of information for this driver?

A) *Rand McNally Road Atlas*
B) *Dubuque Then and Now*
C) *Art of the State: Iowa*
D) *World Atlas for Young Explorers*

36. He gave us a terse reply; he obviously had little time for us.

Which of the following is the definition of the word *terse*?

A) Abrupt
B) Unhelpful
C) Vicious
D) Rhymed

37. Halley's "discovery" of the comet now officially designated as 1P/Halley[1] was not so much a discovery of a new object as an acknowledgment of its recurrence.

What is the purpose of using superscript for the numeral *1* above?

A) To denote the first use of the term
B) To indicate a footnote
C) To explain that this is the primary name
D) To set off the nomenclature

GO ON TO THE NEXT PAGE

38. Opiates are named for the source of their power, the opium found in the poppy known as *Papaver somniferum*. Opium from that poppy contains the analgesics morphine and codeine plus the non-narcotics papaverine, thebaine, and noscapine. Morphine, the most prevalent alkaloid in opium, may be processed chemically (and illegally) to produce heroin. In legal use, morphine is used to treat sudden, overwhelming pain; it must not be used over long periods of time because of its addictive qualities. The 19th-century drug of choice, laudanum, contained most of the opium alkaloids.

A patient presents with chronic back pain. Which opiate might most reasonably be prescribed?

A) Morphine
B) Codeine
C) Thebaine
D) Laudanum

39.

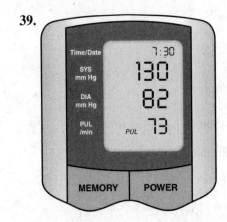

Based on the blood pressure monitor above, which of the following is the patient's diastolic pressure?

A) 73
B) 82
C) 130
D) $\dfrac{130}{82}$

40.

Treatment for	Brand-Name Drug	Generic Drug
High cholesterol	$95/month	$37/month
Arthritis	$135/month	$30/month
Heartburn	$179/month	$15/month

GO ON TO THE NEXT PAGE

Kyle takes an arthritis drug daily. His insurance will only pay for the generic equivalent. How much will Kyle's medication cost per day?

A) About $1 a day
B) About $2 a day
C) About $3 a day
D) About $4 a day

SMOKE DETECTORS 281

SIGN LANGUAGE

See Translators & Interpreters

Di MARCO SIGNS
Specialists in illumination
and backlighting
185 Elm St.

SIGNS

American Sign 15 Morton St 555-1284

Carbon Copies 87 Main St 555-2499

Di Marco Signs 185 Elm St 555-3434

Marshall Signs 24 Main St 555-3100

SKI INSTRUCTION
Bergen Skis Truxton Blvd . . . 555-3116
Donahue Trails 13 Pine Rd . . . 555-9495
SKIN CARE
Altima Spa 425 Morton St . . . 555-6880
Krystal's on Main 23 Main St . . . 555-8300
SMOKE DETECTORS
Alarm Service 280 Elm St . . . 555-2413

SIGNS—ERECTING & HANGING

American Sign 15 Morton St 555-1284

SIGNS—MAINTENANCE & REPAIR

Di Marco Signs 185 Elm St 555-3434

Marshall Signs 24 Main St 555-3100

SKATING RINKS & PARKS

Cass Park Rink 701 Judd Rd 555-9411

JM Sports Complex College Pl . . . .

www.jmcomplex.net 555-1414

KRYSTAL's ON MAIN STREET
Full-service salon
nails, hair, makeup,
spa services

The next two questions are based on this sample yellow page.

41. A customer wants to purchase an illuminated sign for her new café. Which of the following businesses should she call first?

A) American Sign
B) Carbon Copies
C) Di Marco Signs
D) Marshall Signs

42. A café owner wishes to have a new sign hung above her front door. Which number should the owner probably call?

A) 555-1284
B) 555-2499
C) 555-3434
D) 555-3100

GO ON TO THE NEXT PAGE

43.

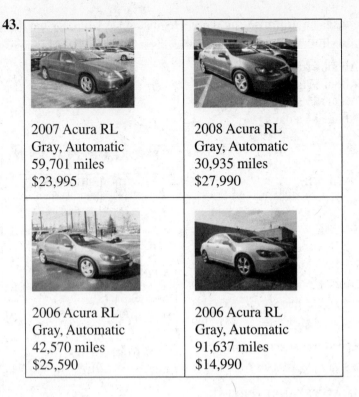

2007 Acura RL Gray, Automatic 59,701 miles $23,995	2008 Acura RL Gray, Automatic 30,935 miles $27,990
2006 Acura RL Gray, Automatic 42,570 miles $25,590	2006 Acura RL Gray, Automatic 91,637 miles $14,990

The pricing of these cars seems primarily to be based on what feature?

A) Model year
B) Mileage
C) Color
D) Model

44. As a <u>paradigm</u> of conservatism run amok, Senator Guthrie has no equal.

Which of the following is the definition of the word *paradigm*?

A) Contradiction
B) Subsection
C) Model
D) Freeloader

GO ON TO THE NEXT PAGE

I attended most of the budget sessions of our local school board this year. Of all the local schools, ours has actually reduced spending. Sadly, due to cuts in state aid, they were not able to reduce the levy significantly. Nevertheless, I hope that all local voters will support the school district's responsible budget. Do not forget to visit the polls on Tuesday, May 13.

The next two questions are based on this passage.

45. Based on the passage, which of the following is a logical prediction of what the author will do?

   A) Vote yes on the school budget
   B) Vote no on the school budget
   C) Attend the district's budget session
   D) Run for a position on the school board

46. Based on a prior knowledge of literature, the reader can infer that this passage was taken from which of the following?

   A) A magazine article
   B) A mystery story
   C) A letter to the editor
   D) A citizenship manual

47. A student planning a presentation wants to open with a memorable line that ties her themes together. Which of the following resources would be most appropriate for her to use?

   A) *Merriam-Webster's Collegiate Dictionary*
   B) *How to Speak and Write Correctly*
   C) *Bartlett's Familiar Quotations*
   D) *PowerPoint Step by Step*

48. Read and follow the directions below.

   1. Imagine 10 blocks: 5 red squares and 5 blue triangles.
   2. Remove 2 blue triangles.
   3. Add 2 red triangles.
   4. Remove 1 red square.
   5. Add 3 blue squares.

   Which of the following describes the blocks now?

   A) 5 triangles, 7 squares
   B) 6 triangles, 6 squares
   C) 7 triangles, 5 squares
   D) 5 triangles, 6 squares

GO ON TO THE NEXT PAGE

Jon Westford <jwestford@gcl.us>

Update   10:45 AM

To: Administrative Staff

I wanted to let everyone know that attendance at Tuesday's workshop, though not mandatory, is highly recommended. Last year's leadership workshop by Management Inc. led to several worthwhile changes in the way we do things at GCL, including our new collaborative goals and action plans. This one, with its emphasis on teamwork, is sure to be equally useful.

MANAGEMENT INC.

Workshops to Enhance Leadership

I. Lead, Don't Lecture

II. Relationships in the Workplace: Building a Winning Team

III. Customer Service & Customer Satisfaction

IV. Making Meetings Meaningful

V. Hiring, Training, and Launching Staff

The next two questions are based on this e-mail and flyer.

49. Which of the Management Inc. workshops will apparently be presented to the administrative staff on Tuesday?

A) Workshop I
B) Workshop II
C) Workshop III
D) Workshop IV

50. What key support does Jon Westford give for his recommendation?

A) He states that attendance is not mandatory.
B) He points out that the workshop is highly recommended.
C) He reminds staff that Management Inc. did a workshop last year.
D) He mentions some changes that came out of last year's workshop.

GO ON TO THE NEXT PAGE

Making Spinach Pesto

The critical ingredients in pesto are olive oil, garlic, pine nuts or other nuts, and Parmesan cheese. The main ingredient can change depending on your whim.

Although most people make pesto from basil, in reality, any leafy green vegetable will do. In fact, I've even had pesto made with asparagus, tomatoes, or squash! But one of my favorites is spinach pesto, because it tastes wonderful and has all the iron that spinach provides. So if you have spinach in your garden, and most of you gardeners do, try this!

Take 2 cups washed and stemmed spinach leaves, ½ cup fresh parsley, ½ cup toasted pine nuts (or try walnuts!), ¼ cup Parmesan cheese, 3 cloves of garlic, 2 tablespoons olive oil, and some salt and pepper. Place everything in a food processor and blend into a paste. You may keep the results in ice cube trays, frozen, and pop them out as you need them.

The next three questions are based on this passage.

51. According to the author, which of the following is a critical ingredient of pesto?

    A) Basil
    B) Olive oil
    C) Pine nuts
    D) Pepper

52. What should you do before putting spinach into the food processor?

    A) Prepare the ice cube trays.
    B) Add parsley and Parmesan cheese.
    C) Separate the leaves from the stems.
    D) Blend the pine nuts with oil and garlic.

53. Which reason does the author give to support her preference for spinach pesto?

    A) It contains iron.
    B) It is a leafy vegetable.
    C) It blends well with garlic.
    D) It grows in most gardens.

STOP. THIS IS THE END OF PART I.

Part II. Mathematics

36 items (32 scored), 54 minutes

1. $3\dfrac{1}{4} \times \dfrac{1}{16}$

Simplify the expression above. Which of the following is correct?

A) $\dfrac{5}{8}$

B) $\dfrac{13}{16}$

C) $\dfrac{13}{64}$

D) $3\dfrac{3}{16}$

2.

City	Population, 2009	Population, 1999
Detroit, Michigan	910,921	965,074
Jacksonville, Florida	813,518	695,877
Memphis, Tennessee	676,640	606,109
San Francisco, California	815,358	747,777

The chart above shows the populations of four cities in two different years.

Which city had the greatest growth between 1999 and 2009?

A) Detroit
B) Jacksonville
C) Memphis
D) San Francisco

GO ON TO THE NEXT PAGE

3.

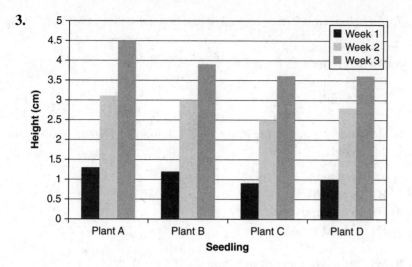

The graph above shows the growth in centimeters of four seedlings.

Which plant showed the least growth between weeks 1 and 3?

A) Plant A
B) Plant B
C) Plant C
D) Plant D

4. Find the total area of the figure shown.

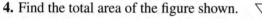

A) 28 cm²
B) 38 cm²
C) 40 cm²
D) 46 cm²

5. $(2x - 1)(x + 5)$

Simplify the expression above. Which of the following is correct?

A) $2x^2 - 5$
B) $2x^2 - 4$
C) $2x^2 - 5x - 5$
D) $2x^2 + 9x - 5$

6. 15 is 20% of what number?

A) 3
B) 45
C) 75
D) 300

GO ON TO THE NEXT PAGE

7. If a train travels 270 miles in 3 hours, how far will it travel in 4.5 hours?

    A) 300 miles
    B) 350 miles
    C) 405 miles
    D) 425 miles

8. How many pounds are there in 8 kilograms? (Note: 1 kilogram = 2.2 pounds.)

    A) 3.6 pounds
    B) 16 pounds
    C) 16.6 pounds
    D) 17.6 pounds

9. What is the product of the numbers 0.35×0.25?

    A) 0.00875
    B) 0.0875
    C) 0.875
    D) 8.75

10. At the bake sale, Josie bought three brownies for $1.35 apiece. She paid with a $5 bill. What change did she receive?

    A) $0.85
    B) $0.95
    C) $1.05
    D) $1.15

11. Angela's scores on five science tests were 85, 82, 94, 96, and 88. What was the average of her test scores?

    A) 87
    B) 88
    C) 89
    D) 90

12. Express 20% as a fraction in lowest terms.

    A) $\dfrac{1}{2}$

    B) $\dfrac{1}{5}$

    C) $\dfrac{1}{10}$

    D) $\dfrac{1}{20}$

GO ON TO THE NEXT PAGE

13. $4\dfrac{1}{8} \div 1\dfrac{1}{2}$

Simplify the expression above. Which of the following is correct?

A) $4\dfrac{1}{2}$

B) $4\dfrac{1}{4}$

C) $2\dfrac{3}{4}$

D) $2\dfrac{1}{4}$

14.

Sodas	$1.75
Chips and Salsa	$2.25
Subs	$3.15
French Fries	$1.25

The concession stand menu above shows the cost of several items.

A customer bought 2 subs, an order of French fries, and 2 sodas. How much did he pay in all?

A) $7.55
B) $9.30
C) $11.05
D) $13.25

GO ON TO THE NEXT PAGE

15.

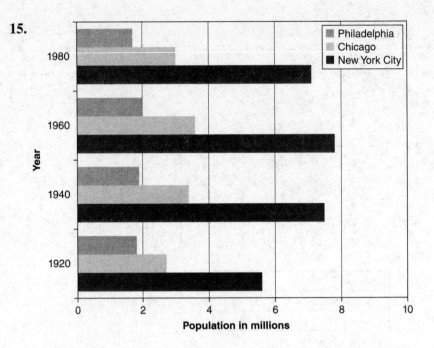

The graph above shows the population of three American cities.

Between which two years did the population of all three cities decline?

A) 1920 and 1940
B) 1940 and 1960
C) 1960 and 1980
D) It never declined in all three cities at once.

16. How many milliliters are there in 4 liters?

A) 40,000 milliliters
B) 4,000 milliliters
C) 400 milliliters
D) 40 milliliters

17. What is the product of 0.52×0.04?

A) 0.00208
B) 0.0208
C) 0.208
D) 2.08

18. The daily average temperatures during one week in July were 70°F, 72°F, 76°F, 69°F, 76°F, 75°F, and 73°F. What was true of the median temperature during that week?

A) It equaled the average temperature.
B) It was the same as the mode.
C) It was less than the average temperature.
D) It was greater than the mode.

GO ON TO THE NEXT PAGE

19. Which of these examples illustrates a positive correlation?

    A) As government spending increased during World War II, consumer spending dropped precipitously.
    B) The increase in consumption by citizens in the 1980s led to a similar rise in the GDP.
    C) The higher the expense ratio of a mutual fund, the lower the investor's returns will be.
    D) As the dollar depreciates against foreign currencies, the value of gold will rise.

20. Which type of graph would best indicate the percentage of a hospital budget spent on various items?

    A) Line graph
    B) Histogram
    C) Circle graph
    D) Scatter plot

21. Order this list of numbers from least to greatest.

$$-2, 2.3, -1.5, \frac{11}{5}$$

A) $-2, -1.5, \frac{11}{5}, 2.3$

B) $-1.5, -2, 2.3, \frac{11}{5}$

C) $-2, -1.5, 2.3, \frac{11}{5}$

D) $-1.5, -2, \frac{11}{5}, 2.3$

22. A number is 10 less than double a given number.

    Translate this phrase into a mathematical expression.

    A) $2n - 10$
    B) $(n + 2) - 10$
    C) $2(n - 10)$
    D) $n - 10 \times 2$

GO ON TO THE NEXT PAGE

23. $|x + 2| = 8$

Which of the following is the solution set for the equation above?

A) $\{6, -6\}$
B) $\{6, -10\}$
C) $\{6, 6\}$
D) $\{-6, 10\}$

24. For a species count, a scientist is measuring the length of a clearing in the forest. Which would be an appropriate unit of measure?

A) Mile
B) Kilometer
C) Meter
D) Centimeter

25. A plan for a house is drawn on a 1:40 scale. If the length of the living room on the plan measures 4.5 inches, what is the actual length of the built living room?

A) 45 feet
B) 25 feet
C) 15 feet
D) 12 feet

26. Grayson left a $2.43 tip for a lunch that cost $13.50. What percent tip did he leave?

A) 16%
B) 18%
C) 20%
D) 22%

27. Find the volume of a box 6 inches high, 6 inches wide, and 6 inches deep.

A) 18 cubic inches
B) 36 cubic inches
C) 128 cubic inches
D) 216 cubic inches

28. How many miles are there in 8 kilometers? (Note: 1 mile = 1.6 kilometers.)

A) 4.6 miles
B) 5 miles
C) 10 miles
D) 12.8 miles

GO ON TO THE NEXT PAGE

29.

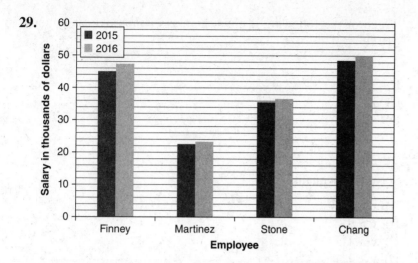

The graph shows the salaries of four employees at Corporation Y.

Employees in the union got a negotiated raise of 3 percent in 2016. Which employee is apparently *not* in the union?

A) Finney
B) Martinez
C) Stone
D) Chang

30. $2\dfrac{3}{5} \times 1\dfrac{1}{8}$

Simplify the expression above. Which of the following is correct?

A) $2\dfrac{37}{40}$

B) $2\dfrac{5}{8}$

C) $2\dfrac{3}{40}$

D) $3\dfrac{1}{20}$

31. Colleen's textbook purchases for the semester come to $55, $69, $74, $40, and $34. Which of the following is an accurate estimate of her textbook expenses?

A) $270
B) $300
C) $320
D) $370

GO ON TO THE NEXT PAGE

32. Which of the following decimal numbers is approximately equal to $\sqrt{10}$?

A) 3.1

B) 3.16

C) 3.2

D) 3.26

33. $3x + 3 > 9$

Solve the inequality.

A) $x > 3$

B) $x > 2$

C) $x > 1$

D) $x \geq 1$

34. Professor Simpson's class has 75 students in all. Thirty of them are women. Which of the following is the ratio of women to the total number of students in the class?

A) $\dfrac{3}{5}$

B) $\dfrac{1}{4}$

C) $\dfrac{2}{3}$

D) $\dfrac{2}{5}$

35. At her nail salon, Rita charges $15 for a manicure and $24 for a pedicure. If on Tuesday, x patrons request manicures, and y patrons request pedicures, what does Rita collect for manicures and pedicures on Tuesday?

A) $\$15x + \$24y$

B) $\$39(x + y)$

C) $\$9(xy)$

D) $(\$15 + x)(\$24 + y)$

GO ON TO THE NEXT PAGE

36. $5x + 3x - 4 = 6x + 2$

Which of the following shows the steps to use to solve for x?

A) $15x - 4 = 6x + 2$
$15x = 6x + 6$
$9x = 6$

B) $3x - 4 = x + 2$
$3x = x + 2$
$2x = 2$

C) $8x - 4 = 6x + 2$
$2x - 4 = 2$
$2x = 6$

D) $5x + 3x + 6x = 2 + 4$
$14x = 6$

STOP. THIS IS THE END OF PART II.

Part III. Science

53 items (47 scored), 63 minutes

1. Which of the following is the function of the cytoskeleton?

   A) Respiration
   B) Storage
   C) Movement
   D) Energy production

2.

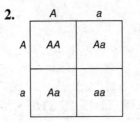

In the diagram above, both parents carry the recessive gene for cystic fibrosis (*a*). Any homozygous recessive offspring will manifest the disease. What percentage of the offspring are predicted to be carriers but not manifest the disease?

   A) 0%
   B) 25%
   C) 50%
   D) 100%

3. What is a sarcomere?

   A) An abnormal collection of inflammatory cells
   B) A typically harmless genus of fungus
   C) One of the ligaments that supports the pelvis
   D) The smallest contractile unit of striated muscle tissue

4. Which is an anterior muscle?

   A) Gluteus maximus
   B) Biceps femoris
   C) Adductor magnus
   D) Quadriceps femoris

5. The lateral side of the right knee would be

   A) the kneecap.
   B) closest to the left knee.
   C) farthest from the left knee.
   D) on the underside of the knee.

GO ON TO THE NEXT PAGE

6. The ovaries are part of the _____ system.

Which of the following completes the sentence above?

A) skeletal
B) nervous
C) lymphatic
D) reproductive

7. The headrest on a car may prevent traumatic injury by limiting

A) hyperflexion of the neck.
B) hyperextension of the neck.
C) vertebral compression.
D) disc degeneration.

8. In a whiplash injury, you might expect to see

A) cardiopulmonary problems.
B) side-to-side spinal curvature.
C) eventual herniation of discs.
D) traumatic injury to ligaments.

9. When a junked car is compacted, which statement is true?

A) Its mass increases.
B) Its mass decreases.
C) Its density increases.
D) Its density decreases.

10. Which is an example of deductive reasoning?

A) Ten of the 100 applicants are left-handed; therefore, 10 percent of the general population must be left-handed.
B) I know several left-handed artists; therefore, left-handed people must have an artistic aptitude.
C) Left-handed people are artistic. Jon is left-handed. Therefore, Jon must be artistic.
D) I see that Jon is left-handed. Jon is a gifted artist. Therefore, left-handed people must be gifted artists.

11. If gas A has four times the molar mass of gas B, you would expect it to diffuse through a plug

A) at half the rate of gas B.
B) at twice the rate of gas B.
C) at a quarter the rate of gas B.
D) at four times the rate of gas B.

GO ON TO THE NEXT PAGE

12. What causes the heart sounds heard through a stethoscope?

A) Closing of valves
B) Turbulence of blood
C) Relaxation of muscles
D) Cardiac output

13. Three students measured the mass of a product of combustion. They recorded measurements of 5.14 g, 5.16 g, and 5.17 g. If the known mass of the product is 5.3 g, the students' measurements were _____.

Which of the following correctly completes the sentence above?

A) accurate
B) precise
C) both accurate and precise
D) neither accurate nor precise

14.

Group	Average Time Taken to Complete 5 km on Treadmill (minutes)	
	Before Consuming Supplements	After Consuming Supplements
1 – Women with iron deficiencies provided with iron supplement	25.5	23.1
2 – Women with iron deficiencies provided with placebo	25.4	25.2

What hypothesis was tested by this experiment?

A) Iron supplements have similar effects on women with and without iron deficiencies.
B) Iron supplements may mask endurance problems in women with iron deficiencies.
C) Women with iron deficiencies can better their performance by taking iron supplements.
D) Women with iron deficiencies perform less well on tasks requiring endurance than women without those deficiencies.

GO ON TO THE NEXT PAGE

15. Where does the digestion of fat mostly take place?

    A) In the liver
    B) In the pancreas
    C) In the large intestine
    D) In the small intestine

16. What causes the pain known as heartburn?

    A) Intrathoracic pressure
    B) Spasms of the esophageal muscle
    C) Hypotension due to depletion of plasma volume
    D) Turbulent flow of blood through narrowed valves

17. Which would *not* be a likely component of a quantitative investigation?

    A) Record keeping
    B) Data management
    C) Graphing data
    D) Interviewing

GO ON TO THE NEXT PAGE

18.

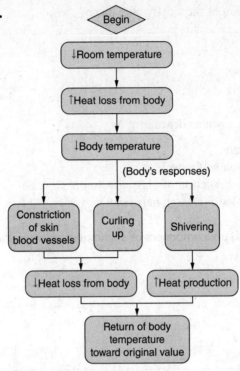

What does this diagram show?

A) Immune response
B) Diffusion
C) Glycolysis
D) Homeostasis

19. Which type of nutrient does not provide the body with energy?

A) Vitamin
B) Carbohydrate
C) Fat
D) Protein

20. Why might certain young people be underweight?

A) They are growing in height faster than they are gaining weight.
B) They eat little protein and too much fat and sugar.
C) They eat several meals a day and fail to exercise enough.
D) They seldom eat a meal that contains foods from all food groups.

GO ON TO THE NEXT PAGE

21. A 20-ml sample of pure gas is enclosed in a glass cylinder at 20°C. If the cylinder is placed in an ice bath at 0°C, what happens to the gas's volume, assuming that the pressure remains constant?

A) It increases.
B) It decreases.
C) It stays the same.
D) It rises, then falls.

22. A student predicts that coffee beans grown in Brazil contain more caffeine than those grown in Nigeria. This prediction corresponds to which of the following steps in the scientific method?

A) Formulating a hypothesis
B) Collecting data
C) Analyzing data
D) Drawing a conclusion

GO ON TO THE NEXT PAGE

23.

PERIODIC TABLE OF THE ELEMENTS

1 H																	2 He
3 Li	4 Be											5 B	6 C	7 N	8 O	9 F	10 Ne
11 Na	12 Mg											13 Al	14 Si	15 P	16 S	17 Ci	18 Ar
19 K	20 Ca	21 Sc	22 Ti	23 V	24 Cr	25 Mn	26 Fe	27 Co	28 Ni	29 Cu	30 Zn	31 Ga	32 Ge	33 As	34 Se	35 Br	36 Kr
37 Rb	38 Sr	39 Y	40 Z	41 Nb	42 Mo	43 Tc	44 Ru	45 Rh	46 Pd	47 Ag	48 Cd	49 In	50 Sn	51 Sb	52 Te	53 I	54 Xe
55 Cs	56 Ba	see below	72 Hf	73 Ta	74 W	75 Re	76 Os	77 It	78 Pt	79 Au	80 Hg	81 Ti	82 Pb	83 Bi	84 Po	85 At	86 Rn
87 Fr	88 Ra	see below	104 Rf	105 Db	106 Sg	107 Bh	108 Hs	109 Mt	110 Ds	111 Rg	112 Uub	113 Uut	114 Uuq	115 Uup	116 Uuh	117 Uus	118 Uuo

■ = Alkali Metals   ■ = Halogens   ■ = Noble Gases

RARE EARTH ELEMENTS

Lanthanides	57 La	58 Ce	59 Pr	60 Nd	61 Pm	62 Sm	63 Eu	64 Gd	65 Tb	66 Dy	67 Ho	68 Er	69 Tm	70 Yb	71 Lu
Actinides	89 Ac	90 Th	91 Pa	92 U	93 Np	94 Pu	95 Am	96 Cm	97 Bk	98 Cf	99 Es	100 Fm	101 Md	102 No	103 Lr

Which of the following elements would you expect to be least reactive?

A) Li
B) Cr
C) Nd
D) Xe

GO ON TO THE NEXT PAGE

24. In which of the following glands is melatonin produced?

A) Pancreas
B) Pituitary
C) Thyroid
D) Pineal

25. Which of the following events might cause a pupillary reflex?

A) Sudden sound
B) Bright light
C) Firm touch
D) High heat

26. Which of the following muscles flexes the elbow joint?

A) Pronator quadratus
B) Palmaris longus
C) Flexor carpi ulnaris
D) Biceps brachii

27. How does the nervous system work with the muscular system?

A) The muscles of the body produce chemicals that feed the nerves.
B) The nervous system releases chemicals that remove excess waste from the muscles.
C) The muscular system provides input that allows the nerves to make decisions.
D) The nervous system tells the muscles how to respond to the environment.

28. In an experiment conducted to compare hours of sleep clocked by male and female freshmen in college, the gender of the freshmen is which type of variable?

A) Dependent
B) Independent
C) Responding
D) Random

GO ON TO THE NEXT PAGE

29. Which organ system is primarily responsible for regulating muscle growth?

   A) The skeletal system
   B) The endocrine system
   C) The nervous system
   D) The reproductive system

30. Which of the following is a floating bone?

   A) Hyoid
   B) Sternum
   C) Sacrum
   D) Coccyx

31. Why doesn't a raindrop accelerate as it approaches the ground?

   A) Gravity pulls it down at a constant rate.
   B) Air resistance balances the gravitational force.
   C) Its mass decreases, decreasing its speed.
   D) Objects in motion decelerate over distance.

32. Which vehicle has the greatest momentum?

   A) A 9,000-kg railroad car traveling at 3 m/s
   B) A 2,000-kg automobile traveling at 24 m/s
   C) A 1,500-kg mini coupe traveling at 29 m/s
   D) A 5,00-kg glider traveling at 89 m/s

33. Which of the following valves allows blood to flow from the right atrium to the right ventricle?

   A) Mitral valve
   B) Aortic valve
   C) Tricuspid valve
   D) Pulmonary valve

34. When a scientist graphed the correlation between the population of a certain species of fish and the temperature of the water in which they lived, she discovered that as the temperature decreased, the population went down. How would you describe this correlation?

   A) Direct
   B) Inverse
   C) Scattered
   D) Logarithmic

GO ON TO THE NEXT PAGE

35. Which of the following would probably *not* be a symptom of aortic stenosis?

A) Anemia
B) Chest pain
C) Breathlessness
D) Fainting

36. The dorsal body cavity is _____ to the ventral body cavity.

Which of the following correctly completes the sentence above?

A) medial
B) deep
C) posterior
D) anterior

37. Which part of the brain is most posterior?

A) Frontal lobe
B) Parietal lobe
C) Temporal lobe
D) Occipital lobe

38. The trachea is part of the _____ system.

Which of the following correctly completes the sentence above?

A) cardiovascular
B) endocrine
C) respiratory
D) digestive

39. Which is a major difference between eukaryotic and prokaryotic cells?

A) Eukaryotes have DNA, and prokaryotes have RNA.
B) Eukaryotes are animal cells, and prokaryotes are plant cells.
C) Eukaryotes have nuclei, and prokaryotes have no nuclei.
D) Eukaryotes house ribosomes, and prokaryotes have no ribosomes.

GO ON TO THE NEXT PAGE

40.

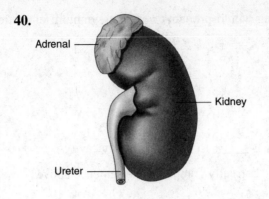

Adrenal

Kidney

Ureter

To what two systems do the pictured body parts belong?

A) Reproductive and endocrine
B) Urinary and reproductive
C) Endocrine and urinary
D) Digestive and cardiovascular

41.

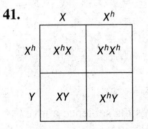

Hemophilia is a sex-linked trait. In the example above of a male with hemophilia and a female carrier, what percentage of the offspring are predicted to be carriers only?

A) 0%
B) 25%
C) 50%
D) 100%

42. One difference between DNA and RNA is that

A) in RNA, adenine bonds with uracil.
B) in RNA, guanine is replaced by adenine.
C) DNA has three bases, whereas RNA has four.
D) DNA lacks the hydrogen bonds found in RNA.

GO ON TO THE NEXT PAGE

43. Which of the following enzymes primarily assists in the digestion of proteins?

A) Maltase
B) Pepsin
C) Amylase
D) Lipase

44. How should a researcher test the hypothesis that practicing yoga reduces blood pressure?

A) Record the blood pressure of one male and one female participant before and after participating in a yoga class.
B) Divide 30 female participants with similar average blood pressure into two groups; test each participant's blood pressure after having her participate in a yoga class.
C) Divide 30 female participants with similar average blood pressure into two groups; have one group watch television for an hour while the other group takes a yoga class, and record each participant's blood pressure after the hour. Repeat daily for two weeks.
D) Start with 15 men and 15 women; have the men watch television for an hour while the women take a yoga class, and record each participant's blood pressure after the hour. Reverse, having the men take a yoga class while the women watch television.

45. Which of the following is a mechanoreceptor that detects blood pressure?

A) Chemoreceptor
B) Baroreceptor
C) Thermoreceptor
D) Nocioreceptor

46. Which of the following might be a symptom of thyroid hyperfunction?

A) Goiter
B) Body weight increase
C) High body temperature
D) Depressed nervous system

47. Where in the body would you find the organ of Corti?

A) Ear
B) Brain
C) Liver
D) Ovary

GO ON TO THE NEXT PAGE

48. Which part of the cell houses the organelles?

   A) Vacuole
   B) Plasmids
   C) Cytoplasm
   D) Cell wall

49. Which stage of mitosis occurs directly after prophase?

   A) Anaphase
   B) Prophase II
   C) Metaphase
   D) Telophase

50. _____ is a form of respiration that takes place without _____.

   Which of the following correctly completes the sentence above?

   A) Fermentation; oxygen
   B) Photosynthesis; carbon dioxide
   C) Metabolism; nitrogen
   D) Diffusion; sugar

51. Which of the following is an example of a hinge joint?

   A) Wrist
   B) Thumb
   C) Elbow
   D) Shoulder

52. Which of the following is *not* an example of connective tissue?

   A) Bone
   B) Cartilage
   C) Blood vessel
   D) Myelin

53. Which of the following is a part of the body's nonspecific defense system?

   A) T cell
   B) B cell
   C) Skin
   D) Antibody

STOP. THIS IS THE END OF PART III.

Part IV. English and Language Usage

28 items (24 scored), 28 minutes

1. Due to his mercurial temperament, Justin did not work well with others.

   What is the simple predicate of this sentence?

   A) temperament
   B) not well
   C) work well with others
   D) did work

2. Which sentence is written correctly?

   A) Because she was uncertain of her abilities, Renee asked for help.
   B) Because she was uncertain of her abilities; Renee asked for help.
   C) Because she was uncertain of her abilities Renee asked for help.
   D) Because she was, uncertain of her abilities, Renee asked for help.

3. Dave came inside. He had a bundle in his arms. I noticed Dave. I ran to help Dave.

   To improve sentence fluency, how could you state the information above in a single sentence?

   A) When I noticed Dave coming inside with a bundle in his arms, I ran to help him.
   B) Dave, coming inside with a bundle in his arms, was noticed and helped by me.
   C) Having noticed Dave coming inside, I ran to help him with a bundle in his arms.
   D) After Dave came inside with a bundle in his arms, I ran to help him, having noticed him.

4. Which sort of writing is likely to be the least formal?

   A) Research report
   B) Text message
   C) Office memo
   D) Wedding invitation

5. In which stage of the writing process would you be likely to use an outline?

   A) Revision
   B) Planning
   C) Citation
   D) Drafting

GO ON TO THE NEXT PAGE

6. Based on the prefix, what does *supramaxillary* mean?

A) Above the jaw
B) Below the jaw
C) Of the jaw
D) At the site of the jaw

7. The hockey team _____ traveling to Albany for the semifinals.

Which of the following correctly completes the sentence above?

A) is
B) are
C) be
D) were

8. Never disregard your feelings in matters of the heart.

What kind of sentence is this?

A) Imperative
B) Interrogative
C) Exclamatory
D) Declarative

9. When the lecture was over, two students _____.

Which of the following correctly completes the sentence above?

A) raise their hands to ask questions
B) raised their hands to ask questions
C) have raised their hands to ask questions
D) are raising their hands to ask questions

10. The counselor expected me to accept her advise without question.

What is the error in this sentence?

A) counselor
B) expected
C) accept
D) advise

GO ON TO THE NEXT PAGE

11. The malefactor was insufficiently punished, in our opinion; instead of receiving a substantial fine, the miscreant was sentenced to a paltry probation.

Which words are redundant in the sentence above?

A) insufficiently, substantial
B) fine, probation
C) substantial, paltry
D) malefactor, miscreant

12. Which sentence is the clearest?

A) Resting in its well-built cage, I admired the lovely parrot.
B) Resting in its well-built cage, the lovely parrot was admired by me.
C) I admired the lovely parrot resting in its well-built cage.
D) I admired in its well-built cage the lovely parrot that was resting.

13. I did not see the open carton of orange juice on the shelf standing with the refrigerator door open.

Which phrase or clause is misplaced in the sentence above?

A) I did not see
B) of orange juice
C) on the shelf
D) standing with the refrigerator door open

14. In which of the following sentences does *engage* mean "attract"?

A) The sororities annually engage in several charitable activities.
B) Did you manage to engage a tutor for the summer?
C) A good grammar lesson must engage the students' attention.
D) The clutch in the old tractor will not engage properly.

15. Do you know whether _____ planning to attend?

Which of the following correctly completes the sentence above?

A) their
B) there
C) they're
D) theire

GO ON TO THE NEXT PAGE

16. Which of the following is an example of a correctly punctuated sentence?

   A) She inquired "How long have you wanted to be a doctor?"
   B) She inquired, How long have you wanted to be a doctor?
   C) She inquired, "How long have you wanted to be a doctor"?
   D) She inquired, "How long have you wanted to be a doctor?"

17. Which of the following is the best definition of the word *biohazard*?

   A) Danger to life
   B) Living dangerously
   C) Scientific danger
   D) Danger to Earth

18. Which of the following is an example of a simple sentence?

   A) The book about stones and gems.
   B) The book about stones and gems that I found on the lower shelf was fascinating.
   C) The book about stones and gems had never caught my eye before last Tuesday.
   D) The book about stones and gems fascinated me, but it irritated my geologist friend.

19. Julia's <u>histrionics</u> failed to make an impression on her hard-hearted professor.

   Which of the following is the meaning of the underlined word above?

   A) accomplishments
   B) daring acts
   C) examinations
   D) emotional behavior

20. Which of the following nouns is written in the correct plural form?

   A) tomatoes
   B) oasises
   C) nuclea
   D) daireys

GO ON TO THE NEXT PAGE

21. Which of the following is an example of third-person point of view?

    A) Jonas and I followed their progress on the Internet.
    B) You would have a hard time convincing anyone of that.
    C) The doctor became a patient when he broke his hip.
    D) "Did you enjoy the movie?" Celia asked us politely.

22. His promotion was not <u>unexpected</u>; it was bound to happen sooner or <u>later</u>.

Which of the following correctly identifies the parts of speech in the underlined portions of the sentence above?

    A) Adverb; adjective
    B) Adjective; adverb
    C) Adjective; adjective
    D) Adverb; adverb

23. Which of the following sentences has correct subject-verb agreement?

    A) Without opening the package, each of us knows what is inside it.
    B) Every one of the team members have the will to win this game.
    C) Anyone with a cell phone are welcome to join the search.
    D) Either José or Martin cover for me when I cannot work.

24. The voting was carefully observed by the poll watchers.

Which of the following changes the sentence above so that it is written in the active rather than in the passive voice?

    A) By the poll watchers, the voting was carefully observed.
    B) The voting by the poll watchers was carefully observed.
    C) The voting was observed carefully by the poll watchers.
    D) The poll watchers carefully observed the voting.

25. Which of the following words is written correctly?

    A) hydro-electric
    B) inter-change
    C) intra-mural
    D) loose-limbed

GO ON TO THE NEXT PAGE

26. I see that _____ nearly eleven—will the restaurant have opened _____ doors?

Which of the following sets of words should be used to fill in the blanks in the sentence above?

A) its; its
B) it's; its
C) it's; it's
D) its; it's

27. Follow these steps to solve the puzzle _____ remove the first letter from each word, replace it with the next letter in the alphabet, and add the same letter to the end of the word.

Which of the following punctuation marks correctly completes the sentence above?

A) ;
B) :
C) -
D) ,

28. When <u>Mr. Doward</u> travels by train, a large entourage accompanies _____.

Which of the following options correctly completes the sentence? The antecedent of the pronoun to be added is underlined.

A) it
B) him
C) them
D) he

STOP. THIS IS THE END OF TEAS PRACTICE TEST 1.

TEAS Practice Test 1: Answer Key

PART I: READING

1. C		19. D		37. B
2. A		20. B		38. B
3. B		21. A		39. B
4. A		22. D		40. A
5. A		23. A		41. C
6. C		24. A		42. A
7. C		25. D		43. B
8. C		26. C		44. C
9. B		27. D		45. A
10. A		28. A		46. C
11. A		29. C		47. C
12. B		30. B		48. A
13. D		31. D		49. B
14. B		32. B		50. D
15. D		33. B		51. B
16. B		34. C		52. C
17. B		35. A		53. A
18. A		36. A		

PART II: MATHEMATICS

1. C		13. C		25. C
2. B		14. C		26. B
3. D		15. C		27. D
4. A		16. B		28. B
5. D		17. B		29. A
6. C		18. A		30. A
7. C		19. B		31. A
8. D		20. C		32. B
9. B		21. A		33. B
10. B		22. A		34. D
11. C		23. B		35. A
12. B		24. C		36. C

PART III: SCIENCE

1. C	19. A	37. D
2. C	20. A	38. C
3. D	21. B	39. C
4. D	22. A	40. C
5. C	23. D	41. B
6. D	24. D	42. A
7. B	25. B	43. B
8. D	26. D	44. C
9. C	27. D	45. B
10. C	28. B	46. C
11. A	29. B	47. A
12. A	30. A	48. C
13. B	31. B	49. C
14. C	32. B	50. A
15. D	33. C	51. C
16. B	34. A	52. D
17. D	35. A	53. C
18. D	36. C	

PART IV: ENGLISH AND LANGUAGE USAGE

1. D	11. D	21. C
2. A	12. C	22. B
3. A	13. D	23. A
4. B	14. C	24. D
5. B	15. C	25. D
6. A	16. D	26. B
7. A	17. A	27. B
8. A	18. C	28. B
9. B	19. D	
10. D	20. A	

TEAS Practice Test 1: Explanatory Answers

PART I: READING

1. (C) The title, "Jason Trains for the Triathlon," represents the main idea of the selection—most of the selection is about that main idea.

2. (A) The narrative is not an autobiography (choice D), nor does it direct or persuade readers (choices C and B). It simply tells a story about a would-be athlete who succeeds.

3. (B) According to the second paragraph, "The people there offered good advice, companionship, and a premade series of running and biking maps." They were welcoming and helpful.

4. (A) Only choice A is something that cannot be proved or tested in some way. It is the speaker's belief, not a fact.

5. (A) Rereading the paragraph should prove that beginning triathletes perform all three tasks, making choice B incorrect. Swimming and bicycling precede running, making choice D incorrect. The inference can be made that beginners do a shorter course, making choice C incorrect and choice A correct.

6. (C) Find the one that could just as easily be part of expository writing rather than narrative writing. Facts about a sport don't necessarily mark a piece as narrative.

7. (C) A summary statement should summarize and present the passage's message. Only statement C does this.

8. (C) The writer's motivation is stated clearly in the final paragraph: "I strongly encourage our planning commission to look toward our existing hamlets and villages as the centers of life in our rural towns." He does not like the current path of the planning commission. There is no support for any of the other choices.

9. (B) The writer refers to "our rural towns" and "our rural nodes," but makes it clear that the latter do not yet exist. He lives in a rural area, but not in a node.

10. (A) Because the writer wishes to spur a group to action, his writing is persuasive.

11. (A) The writer says that nodal development is fine for suburbs and exurbs but not for rural communities.

12. (B) In the third paragraph, the writer compares suburban/exurban nodes to those in rural communities.

13. (D) Look at the sentence, and replace the underlined word with the choices that are given: "Physicians use patch tests to _____ the specific causes of contact dermatitis." Choice D is the only correct choice.

14. (B) Why are doctors using a patch test? They are using a patch test to look for causes of dermatitis.

15. (D) The phrase lists some details about philanthropic projects Ms. Thurston has supported.

16. (B) The paragraph might be part of a speech introducing Ms. Thurston to the public. It does not comment on her life (choice C) other than to praise the good work she has accomplished (choice B).

17. (B) Only Simply Bright lenses are described as "tinted."

18. (A) José wants a daily lens, which limits his choices to EZ on the Eyes and Liqui-Fill. Of those two, EZ on the Eyes is cheaper.

19. (D) Find the line for 80 along the *y*-axis and trace along. All but the bar for 2016 extend beyond that line.

20. (B) The tallest bar is the one for 2014.

21. (A) Start with 52 cards. Subtract 4, and add back 1. Subtract another 4, and add back 1. $52 - 4 + 1 - 4 + 1 = 46$

22. (D) A thesaurus is a book of synonyms.

23. (A) Degrees Celsius are shown on the inner circle on the thermometer. On that scale, the arrow rests between 0 and 5.

24. (A) Kate writes in her first sentence that Don asked her to provide a schedule. She is responding to his request.

25. (D) *Optimal* means "best possible" or "most favorable."

26. (C) Infinitives are discussed on pages 97 and 98. The student should begin on page 97, which is where the term is most likely defined.

27. (D) Broad Street runs east-west along the bottom of the map. If a family turns off Broad Street toward the restaurant, they head north along the drive in the park. They then turn west toward the restaurant.

28. (A) If the entire trail is 2 miles long, the first restroom is clearly found early within the first quarter of that.

29. (C) Certain time words may help you identify the order of events here. The series is about a telephone call, and the only order that makes sense is (C), (B), (A), (D). The narrator made the call before talking to either the clerk or Mr. Holder.

30. (B) Items A to E must all fit within the category of "Game Fish." On the list of choices, only mackerel (choice B) are game fish.

31. (D) Working step by step: *start, tarts, marms, harms.*

32. (B) She might place an ad in the classifieds to sublet her apartment.

33. (B) All of the headings should be languages of the Middle East. Yoruba is a language of West Africa.

34. (C) The closer a source is to the actual event, the more likely it is to be a primary source. Articles (choice A), guidebooks (choice B), and reprinted photographs (choice D) are steps removed from the event itself, but contemporaneous hospital records would be primary sources.

35. (A) The road atlas would best help a driver wishing to find a route between these two cities in Iowa.

36. (A) If you speak in a terse manner, you speak abruptly or curtly.

37. (B) Superscript numbers are usually used in expository text to indicate the use of a footnote.

38. (B) If the person has chronic back pain, he or she needs a pain medication that can be taken for a long period of time. That precludes the use of morphine (choice A), which is very addictive. Thebaine (choice C) and noscapine (choice D) are described as non-narcotic. Only codeine (choice B) seems to be a painkiller that might be used for chronic pain.

39. (B) The diastolic pressure is indicated next to the abbreviation *DIA*.

40. (A) Find the row with treatments for arthritis and the column for generic drugs. The generic drug for arthritis will cost about $30 per month, or around $1 per day.

41. (C) DiMarco Signs has an ad in the right column that indicates a specialty in illuminated and backlit signs.

42. (A) Only one listing is given for erecting and hanging signs—American Sign Company, at 555-1284.

43. (B) All of the cars are the same color (choice C), and all are the same model (D) so neither of those is a predictor of price. The model year (choice A) might have to do with the price, but two cars have the same year but very different mileage, and the 2007 car with more miles than the 2006 car costs less. Mileage is clearly the most important variable in determining price.

44. (C) Only the word *model* makes sense in context.

45. (A) The writer hopes "that all local voters will support the school district's responsible budget." It is not a stretch to predict that the writer will vote yes on the budget.

46. (C) This sort of appeal to the public is typical of letters to the editor.

47. (C) Memorable lines to use in speeches or reports may often be found in books of quotations.

48. (A) In problems of this kind, it may help to draw a picture. You start with five red squares and five blue triangles. After step 2, you have five red squares and three blue triangles. After step 3, you have five red squares, three blue triangles, and two red triangles. After step 4, you have four red squares, three blue triangles, and two red triangles. After step 5, you have four red squares, three blue squares (for a total of seven squares), three blue triangles, and two red triangles (for a total of five triangles).

49. (B) The e-mail suggests that the workshop has an "emphasis on team-work." The only workshop listed on the flyer that has such an emphasis is Workshop II, Relationships in the Workplace: Building a Winning Team.

50. (D) Although choices A, B, and C are all true, none of them provides solid support for Jon Westford's recommendation. The fact that the last workshop led to substantive changes (choice D) is evidence that supports his suggestion that this year's workshop will be useful as well.

51. (B) The critical ingredients are listed in the opening sentence. Pine nuts (choice C) are on that list, but the author indicates that other substitutions will do just as well. Of the choices, only olive oil (choice B) is always necessary.

52. (C) Paragraph 3 refers to "washed and stemmed" spinach leaves, meaning that the stems should be removed before the leaves are placed in the food processor.

53. (A) The clue word *because* helps indicate the author's reasoning. She likes spinach pesto because "it tastes wonderful and has all the iron that spinach provides." The best answer is choice A.

Part II: Mathematics

1. (C) To multiply mixed numbers and fractions, first express mixed numbers as fractions. In this case, $3\frac{1}{4}$ may be expressed as $\frac{13}{4}$. Next, multiply numerators and denominators. $13 \times 1 = 13$, and $4 \times 16 = 64$. The answer is $\frac{13}{64}$.

2. (B) Detroit's population declined between the 2 years given. You may estimate the difference of the other cities' populations if you don't wish to work out the subtraction—only Jacksonville increased by more than 100,000 inhabitants.

3. (D) Again, you need not work out the subtraction here—simply looking at the bars and estimating should be enough to show that plant D grew the least.

4. (A) Find the area of the square: 4 cm × 4 cm, or 16 sq cm. Now find the area of the two triangles and add it to that of the square. Both are 3-4-5 right triangles, so you can express their combined area as $2(\frac{1}{2} \times 3$ cm $\times 4$ cm$)$, or twice $\frac{1}{2}bh$. Adding 12 sq cm to 16 sq cm equals 28 sq cm.

5. (D) Start by multiplying the variables: $2x \times x = 2x^2$. Now multiply $2x \times 5$ and $x \times -1$, for $10x - 1x$, or $9x$ in all. Finally, multiply the final digits: 5×-1, equaling -5. The solution is $2x^2 + 9x - 5$.

6. (C) Think: $0.20x = 15$. Solve: $x = 15 \div 0.20$. The answer is 75.

7. (C) Set this up as a proportion: $\frac{270}{3} = \frac{x}{4.5}$. You may cross-multiply to solve: $270 \times 4.5 = 3x$. $1215 = 3x$. $x = \frac{1,215}{3}$, or 405.

8. (D) If 1 kilogram equals 2.2 pounds, 8 kilograms equals 2.2×8, or 17.6 pounds.

9. (B) Multiplying two numbers with two digits to the right of the decimal point should result in a product with four digits to the right of the decimal point.

10. (B) First, determine how much Josie spent: $1.35 × 3 = $4.05. Then subtract that total from $5.00: $5.00 − $4.05 = $0.95.

11. (C) To find the average, add the test scores and divide by the number of test scores: 85 + 82 + 94 + 96 + 88 = 445. 445 ÷ 5 = 89.

12. (B) 20% is the same as $\dfrac{20}{100}$. Reduce that to lowest terms by dividing numerator and denominator by 20: $\dfrac{1}{5}$.

13. (C) Begin by expressing the mixed numbers as improper fractions: $4\dfrac{1}{8} = \dfrac{33}{8}$, and $1\dfrac{1}{2} = \dfrac{3}{2}$. To divide by a fraction, multiply by its reciprocal. Therefore, $\dfrac{33}{8} \div \dfrac{3}{2} = \dfrac{33}{8} \times \dfrac{2}{3}$, or $\dfrac{66}{24}$. Now reduce to lowest terms: $\dfrac{66}{24} \div \dfrac{6}{6} = \dfrac{11}{4}$. Finally, express $\dfrac{11}{4}$ as a mixed number: $2\dfrac{3}{4}$.

14. (C) Express the purchases as an equation: 2($3.15) + $1.25 + 2($1.75) = total. Then solve: $6.30 + $1.25 + $3.50 = total; $11.05 = total.

15. (C) Notice how the dates are listed along the *y*-axis. Between 1920 and 1940 (choice A) and between 1940 and 1960 (choice B), the populations in all three cities grew. Between 1960 and 1980 (choice C), all three populations declined.

16. (B) One liter = 1,000 milliliters, so 4 liters = 4,000 milliliters.

17. (B) Without doing the calculation, you should know that multiplying two numbers with two digits to the right of the decimal point should result in a product with four digits to the right of the decimal point.

18. (A) The median temperature is the middle temperature when all the temperatures are arranged from least to greatest: 69°F, 70°F, 72°F, 73°F, 75°F, 76°F, 76°F. The mode is the most frequent temperature; in this case, 76°F. Knowing that eliminates choices A and C. The average is the sum of the temperatures divided by the number of temperatures: $\dfrac{69 + 70 + 72 + 73 + 75 + 76 + 76}{7}$, or $\dfrac{511}{7}$, or 73°F—precisely equal to the median.

19. (B) In a positive correlation, both variables move in the same direction. If one increases, so does the other. If one decreases, so does the other. Only choice B illustrates this movement: consumption increases, and so does GDP.

20. (C) A circle graph is appropriate for dividing 100 percent into segments.

21. (A) −2 is less than −1.5, and $\dfrac{11}{5}$ = 2.2.

22. (A) If *n* = the given number, doubling it is 2*n*. To find the number that is 10 less, subtract 10 from 2*n*.

23. (B) The bars mean "absolute value," which denotes the distance from zero on the number line and is always expressed as a positive number. It should be easy to find the positive value that added to 2 makes 8. In addition, $-10 + 2 = -8$, and the absolute value of -8 is 8.

24. (C) It would have to be a truly gigantic field for choice A or B to be appropriate, and measuring in centimeters (choice D) would be difficult and not terribly useful. In questions such as this, choose the measurement that is most likely.

25. (C) You can find the answer by setting up a proportion: $\dfrac{1}{40} = \dfrac{4.5}{x}$. Cross-multiplication leads to $x = 4.5(40)$, or $x = 180$ inches. Converting that to feet gets you an answer of $\dfrac{180}{12}$, or 15 feet.

26. (B) To find the percentage that $2.43 is of $13.50, simply divide $2.43 ÷ $13.50. The answer is 0.18, or 18%.

27. (D) Volume is height times width times depth: $6 \times 6 \times 6 = 216$.

28. (B) You might set this up as a proportion: $\dfrac{1}{1.6} = \dfrac{x}{8}$. Solve by cross-multiplying $1.6x = 8$, so $x = \dfrac{8}{1.6}$, or 5.

29. (A) Instead of struggling through the computation, simply look for a difference between the heights of the bars that seems not to be in proportion. Employee Finney seems to have the greatest gap between pay in 2015 and 2016, so the odds are that Finney is not in the union.

30. (A) Express the mixed numbers as improper fractions: $\dfrac{13}{5} \times \dfrac{9}{8}$. Then multiply numerators and denominators for a product of $\dfrac{117}{40}$. Finally, express this as a mixed number in lowest terms: $2\dfrac{37}{40}$.

31. (A) Rounding the numbers to the nearest ten can help you to estimate accurately: $60 + $70 + $70 + $40 + $30 = $270. You can check by performing the actual addition if you have time: $55 + $69 + $74 + $40 + $34 = $272. Your estimate is pretty close!

32. (B) You may wish to solve this by trial and error. Work the easiest ones first; $3.1^2 = 9.61$, which is not terribly close. $3.2^2 = 10.24$. Your answer is likely to be the one in the middle; in fact, $3.16^2 = 9.9856$.

33. (B) You may solve this by trial and error, or you may work it out algebraically: $3x + 3 > 9$; $3x > 6$, so $x > 2$.

34. (D) There are 30 women in a class of 75, so the ratio of women to total membership is $\dfrac{30}{75}$, or, in lowest terms, $\dfrac{2}{5}$.

35. (A) $15x represents the income from manicures, and $24y represents the income from pedicures. Adding the two gives you Rita's income from manicures and pedicures on Tuesday.

36. (C) You may add the x variables on one side of the equation to simplify and then subtract equal amounts of x from both sides of the equation. The last step before solving should involve getting x on one side and a number on the other side. The solution for x is 3. If you are unsure, plug the solution back into the original equation:

$$5(3) + 3(3) - 4 = 6(3) + 2$$
$$15 + 9 - 4 = 18 + 2$$
$$20 = 20$$

Part III: Science

1. (C) The cytoskeleton is a system of fibers and microtubules within a cell that gives the cell shape and enables movement.

2. (C) The gene for the disease is recessive, so only homozygous recessive offspring (aa) manifest the disease. An offspring that carries the recessive gene along with the dominant A gene (Aa) will carry but not manifest the disease.

3. (D) Muscle fibers are made up of myofibrils, which are in turn made up of bands of sarcomeres. Sarcomeres are composed of proteins, including myosin and actin.

4. (D) An anterior muscle is located near the front of the body. Of those listed, the quadriceps (frontal thigh muscle) is the most anterior.

5. (C) Something that is lateral is toward the outer side of the body. The side of the right knee farthest from the left knee would fit this description.

6. (D) The ovaries are the egg-producing reproductive organs.

7. (B) The headrest prevents the head from moving too far backward, or hyperextending the neck beyond its normal range.

8. (D) Because of the hyperflexion and hyperextension caused by such a collision, it is not uncommon to find tears or stretching of the ligaments of the spine. The injury is front-to-back, making choice B unlikely, and a herniated disc (choice C) is more of a compression injury.

9. (C) Since density = mass/volume, it should be obvious that the decrease in volume as a car is crushed should lead to an increase in density. Nothing happens to change the mass of the car.

10. (C) In deductive reasoning, a hypothesis follows from a set of premises. The premises may be true, in which case the reasoning is sound, or they may be untrue or at least dubious, as in this example.

11. (A) Set up a simple equation if it helps. Suppose that gas A has a molar mass of M_1, and gas B has a molar mass four times that, M_2. Now suppose that $M_1 = 1$ and $M_2 = 4$. The square root of $\frac{4}{1} = \frac{2}{1}$, so the rate of effusion for gas A is half that of gas B.

12. (A) The low-pitched sound comes from the closure of the atrioventricular valves at the onset of systole, the phase when the heart muscle pumps blood from the chambers into the arteries. The high-pitched sound comes from the closure of pulmonary and aortic valves at the onset of diastole, the phase when the heart muscle relaxes, enabling the chambers to fill with blood again.

13. (B) The students' measurements were precise, in that they corresponded closely with one another. However, since the true measurement differed from theirs by at least 0.13 gram, the measurements were not terribly accurate.

14. (C) Only women with iron deficiencies were tested, making choices A and D incorrect. The experiment tested rate rather than endurance, making choice B unlikely. The best answer is choice C.

15. (D) Bile, produced in the liver and stored in the gallbladder, is released into the bile duct, just as the pancreas releases lipases, the enzymes that break down fat. Both bile and lipases break down the fat in the small intestine, with the bile salts breaking up large droplets of lipid into smaller particles that combine with fatty acids and 2-monoglycerides produced by the actions of the lipases.

16. (B) Although heartburn appears to occur in the region surrounding the heart, it actually takes place in the esophagus, either when acid is refluxed upward from the stomach or when acid burns the esophageal wall directly as it passes downward.

17. (D) Choices A, B, and C are definitely quantitative, but choice D may or may not be.

18. (D) Homeostasis is the ability of a system or organism to regulate its internal environment to maintain equilibrium. The diagram details the body's response to an external decrease in temperature.

19. (A) Some nutrients supply energy, and others support metabolism. Nutrients in the first set include carbohydrates, proteins, and fats. Those in the second set include vitamins, minerals, and water.

20. (A) This is a common cause of being underweight in adolescents. Choices B and C would more likely lead to being overweight.

21. (B) If the temperature of a gas is decreased at a constant pressure, its volume decreases.

22. (A) Making a prediction that is to be tested is part of the formulation of a hypothesis.

23. (D) Reactivity is the tendency of an element to undergo chemical change, which in turn depends on its stability. Xenon, a noble gas, is extremely stable and thus nonreactive under normal conditions.

24. (D) The small pineal gland in the brain secretes melatonin, which regulates sleep.

25. (B) The pupillary reflex is the dilation of the pupil in response to light falling on the retinal ganglion cells of the eye.

26. (D) The biceps brachii is a two-part muscle extending from the scapula along the upper arm to the humerus and radius. It is a flexor muscle that aids in the bending of the elbow joint. Of the other possible responses, choices B and C help flex the wrist, and choice A helps rotate the arm.

27. (D) The nervous system is made up of the brain, spinal cord, and nerves. It receives and transmits signals from the environment that regulate voluntary and involuntary movement.

28. (B) The dependent variable (choice A) is the one that is affected by the independent variable (choice B). In this case, the gender of the subjects is not affected by the hours of sleep, but the sleep patterns may be affected by the gender of the subjects.

29. (B) Hormones from the endocrine system, particularly from the pituitary gland, regulate growth.

30. (A) The hyoid, found just inferior to the mandible, or jawbone, is the only bone in the body that is not connected to other bones by muscles or ligaments. Thus, it is called a "floating" bone, although it is actually held in place by muscle tissue. It supports the tongue and holds the trachea open.

31. (B) Gravity in fact causes acceleration, making choice A incorrect—unless air resistance counteracts that acceleration, which it may easily do for an object as small and lightweight as a raindrop. Raindrops may lose mass (choice C), but that would not decrease their acceleration. Choice D violates Newton's first law of motion.

32. (B) Momentum is the product of velocity and mass, and the greatest product of the four presented here is 48,000 kg·m/s.

33. (C) The tricuspid valve opens to let blood flow from the top right chamber of the heart to the lower right chamber of the heart. Of the other choices, the mitral valve (choice A) lets blood flow from the left atrium to the left ventricle, the aortic valve (choice B) lets blood flow from the left ventricle to the aorta, and the pulmonary valve (choice D) lets blood flow from the right ventricle through the pulmonary artery.

34. (A) If large values of one variable match large values of the other, and small values of the first variable match small values of the other, the correlation is direct, whether the values increase or decrease.

35. (A) Anemia is a common blood disorder in which the red blood cells do not function correctly or are not sufficient for bodily needs. It is unlikely to be a symptom of aortic stenosis, in which the aortic valve narrows, obstructing blood flow. Typical symptoms range from fatigue and weakness to those symptoms listed in choices B, C, and D.

36. (C) The dorsal body cavity contains the spinal column, making it posterior, or toward the back of the body, compared to the ventral body cavity, which contains the structures of the chest and abdomen.

37. (D) The occipital lobe is farthest back in the skull, posterior to the other parts of the brain.

38. (C) The trachea, or windpipe, filters the air we breathe and funnels it into the bronchi.

39. (C) A good way to remember this is to know that *karyose*, meaning "kernel," is used to refer to the nucleus of a cell. *Pro-* means "before," and *eu-* means "true." So eukaryotes have a true nucleus, and prokaryotes are supposedly an earlier form of cells, ones with no nucleus.

40. (C) The kidney and ureter are part of the urinary tract, and the adrenal gland is part of the endocrine system.

41. (B) Reading the chart clockwise from top left, the cross is predicted to yield one female carrier, one female hemophiliac, one male hemophiliac, and one normal male who neither carries nor manifests the disease. Only one of the four, a female X^hX, is a carrier only.

42. (A) As the DNA molecule is translated into RNA, the pairing of bases changes. Adenine (A) no longer pairs with thymine (T), but rather with uracil (U).

43. (B) Pepsin is a protease, or an enzyme that breaks down the peptide bonds of protein molecules. Of the other responses shown, maltase (choice A) breaks down disaccharide maltose into simple sugar glucose, amylase (choice C) breaks down carbohydrates, and lipase (choice D) breaks down fats.

44. (C) Although it may be useful to compare men and women in a later study (D), the study in choice C does a good job of comparing yoga to another activity over a reasonable period of time.

45. (B) Both baroreceptors (choice B) and nocioreceptors (choice D) are mechanoreceptors (sensory receptors that respond to mechanical energy). Baroreceptors detect blood pressure, and nocioreceptors detect pain. The other choices detect chemical energy (choice A) and heat energy (choice C).

46. (C) Hyperfunction is abnormally increased function. When the thyroid is hyperfunctional, metabolic rates increase, leading to a high body temperature and hyperexcitability of the nervous system. The other choices here are symptoms of hypofunction in the thyroid.

47. (A) The organ of Corti is a receptor organ in the cochlea of the inner ear whose purpose is to extract and transduce sound energy.

48. (C) An organelle is any differentiated structure within the cell; examples include the vacuoles and the mitochondria. All are located within the cytoplasm, that liquid portion within the cell membrane.

49. (C) Prophase II (choice B) is a stage of meiosis. In order, the stages of mitosis are prophase, metaphase, anaphase, and telophase.

50. (A) Fermentation is the anaerobic breakdown of sugar into alcohol.

51. (C) The elbow is a hinge joint in that it allows extension and flexion along a single plane. Of the other examples, the wrist (choice A) is a condyloid joint (and the carpals of the wrist are gliding joints), the thumb (choice B) is a saddle joint, and the shoulder (choice D) is a ball-and-socket joint.

52. (D) Cartilage, tendons, and ligaments are composed of connective tissue, and blood vessels include connective, epithelial, and muscle tissue. Myelin is made of nervous tissue.

53. (C) If it is nonspecific, it does not distinguish among invading organisms. The skin and inflammatory responses are nonspecific.

Part IV: English and Language Usage

1. (D) The simple predicate is the verb in the sentence. In this case, it is a main verb and helping verb—*did work*.

2. (A) This question tests your knowledge of basic punctuation. A comma must appear between the dependent clause *Because she was uncertain of her abilities* and the independent clause *Renee asked for help.* No other commas are needed.

3. (A) Reading the choices aloud may help you determine which choice has a logical order of phrases and clauses. Choice B is passive rather than active, and the other choices misplace certain modifiers.

4. (B) Text messages may include slang or colloquialisms and may not even be punctuated or capitalized correctly.

5. (B) An outline is a graphic organizer designed to help a writer visualize and structure a piece of writing.

6. (A) The prefix *supra-* means "above," so something that is *supramaxillary* appears above the lower jaw.

7. (A) The team is traveling as a unit, making the singular form of the verb correct here.

8. (A) An imperative sentence gives a command or makes a request, and it often contains no visible subject. The subject here is understood to be *you*.

9. (B) In this type of question, you must make sure that the tense of verbs remains consistent. Because *was* is past tense, the correct answer contains another past-tense verb, *raised*.

10. (D) There are several frequently confused words in this sentence, but only *advise* (choice D) is incorrect. The correct word would be *advice*, meaning "recommendation" or "guidance."

11. (D) When in doubt with this kind of question, look for the words that are synonyms. The only synonym pair here is in choice D.

12. (C) Choice A misplaces the modifier, making it seem as though I were resting in a cage. Choice B is passive. Choice D is just confusing. The best choice is C.

13. (D) In questions like this one, try to find the phrase that, if moved around, would improve the sentence. In this case, *Standing with the refrigerator door open* should really begin the sentence. If it did, all phrases would appear properly next to the nouns that they modify.

14. (C) *Engage* has a variety of meanings; among them are "to participate" (choice A), "reserve in advance" (choice B), and "move into position" (choice D). In choice C, to "engage" someone's attention is the same as to attract or capture that person's attention.

15. (C) The sentence could also read: "Do you know whether they are planning to attend?" The contraction means "they are."

16. (D) The quotation is a question. It must be introduced with a comma and contain the question mark within the quotation marks.

17. (A) The root *bio*, as in *biology,* means "life," which should be enough for you to determine the correct definition.

18. (C) A simple sentence has just one subject and verb. Choice A has no verb at all and cannot be called a sentence. Choice B is a complex sentence that contains a dependent clause. Choice D is a compound sentence; it contains two independent clauses.

19. (D) *Histrionics*, from a Latin word for "actor," implies overacting.

20. (A) *Tomatoes* (choice A) is correct. The correct spelling of the other plurals would be *oases, nuclei,* and *dairies.*

21. (C) Third-person pronouns include *it, he, she,* and *they.* Choices A and D are in the first person, and choice B is in the second person.

22. (B) *Unexpected* modifies *promotion*, which is a noun. *Later* modifies *to happen,* which is a verb.

23. (A) The subjects in sentences B and C are *one* and *anyone,* which are singular and require singular forms of verbs. The *either/or* construction in sentence D calls for the verb to agree with the closer of the two subjects. The sentence that is correct (choice A) contains a singular subject, *each,* which is matched properly to a singular form of the verb.

24. (D) Active voice expresses an action performed by a subject rather than an action performed on a subject. The only sentence that follows this rule is choice D.

25. (D) Choices A, B, and C are all closed compounds that require no hyphenation.

26. (B) *It's* means "it is." *Its* means "belonging to it."

27. (B) The clues are "these steps" and the list that follows that introduction. A colon should introduce the list of steps.

28. (B) *Mr. Doward* is the antecedent, and the pronoun must be an object pronoun, not a subject pronoun. Only the word *him* (choice B) fits the sentence.

TEAS PRACTICE TEST 2

TEAS Practice Test 2: Answer Sheet

READING

1 (A) (B) (C) (D)	19 (A) (B) (C) (D)	37 (A) (B) (C) (D)
2 (A) (B) (C) (D)	20 (A) (B) (C) (D)	38 (A) (B) (C) (D)
3 (A) (B) (C) (D)	21 (A) (B) (C) (D)	39 (A) (B) (C) (D)
4 (A) (B) (C) (D)	22 (A) (B) (C) (D)	40 (A) (B) (C) (D)
5 (A) (B) (C) (D)	23 (A) (B) (C) (D)	41 (A) (B) (C) (D)
6 (A) (B) (C) (D)	24 (A) (B) (C) (D)	42 (A) (B) (C) (D)
7 (A) (B) (C) (D)	25 (A) (B) (C) (D)	43 (A) (B) (C) (D)
8 (A) (B) (C) (D)	26 (A) (B) (C) (D)	44 (A) (B) (C) (D)
9 (A) (B) (C) (D)	27 (A) (B) (C) (D)	45 (A) (B) (C) (D)
10 (A) (B) (C) (D)	28 (A) (B) (C) (D)	46 (A) (B) (C) (D)
11 (A) (B) (C) (D)	29 (A) (B) (C) (D)	47 (A) (B) (C) (D)
12 (A) (B) (C) (D)	30 (A) (B) (C) (D)	48 (A) (B) (C) (D)
13 (A) (B) (C) (D)	31 (A) (B) (C) (D)	49 (A) (B) (C) (D)
14 (A) (B) (C) (D)	32 (A) (B) (C) (D)	50 (A) (B) (C) (D)
15 (A) (B) (C) (D)	33 (A) (B) (C) (D)	51 (A) (B) (C) (D)
16 (A) (B) (C) (D)	34 (A) (B) (C) (D)	52 (A) (B) (C) (D)
17 (A) (B) (C) (D)	35 (A) (B) (C) (D)	53 (A) (B) (C) (D)
18 (A) (B) (C) (D)	36 (A) (B) (C) (D)	

MATHEMATICS

1 (A) (B) (C) (D)	13 (A) (B) (C) (D)	25 (A) (B) (C) (D)
2 (A) (B) (C) (D)	14 (A) (B) (C) (D)	26 (A) (B) (C) (D)
3 (A) (B) (C) (D)	15 (A) (B) (C) (D)	27 (A) (B) (C) (D)
4 (A) (B) (C) (D)	16 (A) (B) (C) (D)	28 (A) (B) (C) (D)
5 (A) (B) (C) (D)	17 (A) (B) (C) (D)	29 (A) (B) (C) (D)
6 (A) (B) (C) (D)	18 (A) (B) (C) (D)	30 (A) (B) (C) (D)
7 (A) (B) (C) (D)	19 (A) (B) (C) (D)	31 (A) (B) (C) (D)
8 (A) (B) (C) (D)	20 (A) (B) (C) (D)	32 (A) (B) (C) (D)
9 (A) (B) (C) (D)	21 (A) (B) (C) (D)	33 (A) (B) (C) (D)
10 (A) (B) (C) (D)	22 (A) (B) (C) (D)	34 (A) (B) (C) (D)
11 (A) (B) (C) (D)	23 (A) (B) (C) (D)	35 (A) (B) (C) (D)
12 (A) (B) (C) (D)	24 (A) (B) (C) (D)	36 (A) (B) (C) (D)

SCIENCE

1 (A) (B) (C) (D)   19 (A) (B) (C) (D)   37 (A) (B) (C) (D)
2 (A) (B) (C) (D)   20 (A) (B) (C) (D)   38 (A) (B) (C) (D)
3 (A) (B) (C) (D)   21 (A) (B) (C) (D)   39 (A) (B) (C) (D)
4 (A) (B) (C) (D)   22 (A) (B) (C) (D)   40 (A) (B) (C) (D)
5 (A) (B) (C) (D)   23 (A) (B) (C) (D)   41 (A) (B) (C) (D)
6 (A) (B) (C) (D)   24 (A) (B) (C) (D)   42 (A) (B) (C) (D)
7 (A) (B) (C) (D)   25 (A) (B) (C) (D)   43 (A) (B) (C) (D)
8 (A) (B) (C) (D)   26 (A) (B) (C) (D)   44 (A) (B) (C) (D)
9 (A) (B) (C) (D)   27 (A) (B) (C) (D)   45 (A) (B) (C) (D)
10 (A) (B) (C) (D)   28 (A) (B) (C) (D)   46 (A) (B) (C) (D)
11 (A) (B) (C) (D)   29 (A) (B) (C) (D)   47 (A) (B) (C) (D)
12 (A) (B) (C) (D)   30 (A) (B) (C) (D)   48 (A) (B) (C) (D)
13 (A) (B) (C) (D)   31 (A) (B) (C) (D)   49 (A) (B) (C) (D)
14 (A) (B) (C) (D)   32 (A) (B) (C) (D)   50 (A) (B) (C) (D)
15 (A) (B) (C) (D)   33 (A) (B) (C) (D)   51 (A) (B) (C) (D)
16 (A) (B) (C) (D)   34 (A) (B) (C) (D)   52 (A) (B) (C) (D)
17 (A) (B) (C) (D)   35 (A) (B) (C) (D)   53 (A) (B) (C) (D)
18 (A) (B) (C) (D)   36 (A) (B) (C) (D)

ENGLISH AND LANGUAGE USAGE

1 (A) (B) (C) (D)   11 (A) (B) (C) (D)   21 (A) (B) (C) (D)
2 (A) (B) (C) (D)   12 (A) (B) (C) (D)   22 (A) (B) (C) (D)
3 (A) (B) (C) (D)   13 (A) (B) (C) (D)   23 (A) (B) (C) (D)
4 (A) (B) (C) (D)   14 (A) (B) (C) (D)   24 (A) (B) (C) (D)
5 (A) (B) (C) (D)   15 (A) (B) (C) (D)   25 (A) (B) (C) (D)
6 (A) (B) (C) (D)   16 (A) (B) (C) (D)   26 (A) (B) (C) (D)
7 (A) (B) (C) (D)   17 (A) (B) (C) (D)   27 (A) (B) (C) (D)
8 (A) (B) (C) (D)   18 (A) (B) (C) (D)   28 (A) (B) (C) (D)
9 (A) (B) (C) (D)   19 (A) (B) (C) (D)
10 (A) (B) (C) (D)   20 (A) (B) (C) (D)

Part I. Reading

53 questions (47 scored), 64 minutes

The World War II Museum

The National World War II Museum began as the D-Day Museum. Founded by historian Stephen Ambrose to celebrate the amphibious invasions of World War II, the museum has morphed over time into a fascinating and user-friendly exploration of the wars in Europe and the Pacific. In the future, it will include a pavilion with restored torpedo boats and a large center that includes a restored Flying Fortress aircraft. The final section of the campus will be the Liberation Pavilion, an in-depth examination of the Holocaust.

Veterans of World War II are invited to sign the Roll of Honor as they enter the museum, and many special events for veterans are held throughout the year. The main building houses exhibitions on the Pacific Theater and the Home Front on the second floor, and the Normandy Invasion and the European Theater on the third floor. Across the street is a complex featuring a theater, museum store, and two restaurants.

The museum is open seven days a week from 9 A.M. until 5 P.M. It is closed on Mardi Gras Day, Thanksgiving Day, Christmas Eve, and Christmas Day. Documentaries are shown daily on the half-hour from 9:30 A.M. until 3:30 P.M.

The next five questions are based on this passage.

1. The reader can infer that this passage was taken from which of the following?

   A) An encyclopedia
   B) A history textbook
   C) A tourist brochure
   D) A World War II novel

2. The description of the growth of the museum in the first paragraph is reflective of which of the following types of text structure?

   A) Sequence
   B) Cause-effect
   C) Problem-solution
   D) Comparison-contrast

3. The author intends to do which of the following by using the words "fascinating and user-friendly exploration"?

   A) Persuade
   B) Inform
   C) Entertain
   D) Reflect

GO ON TO THE NEXT PAGE

4. Which of the following conclusions may be drawn directly from the third paragraph of the passage?

    A) You could visit the museum on a Sunday afternoon.
    B) You could see a documentary at 4 P.M. on Tuesday.
    C) Mardi Gras Day is not a holiday at the museum.
    D) The museum is open to the public every weeknight.

5. The passage reflects which of the following types of writing?

    A) Narrative story
    B) Expository essay
    C) Technical manual
    D) Persuasive speech

The School Calendar

The school calendar for Dryden School District, like most school calendars, is crammed with concerts and sporting events. There are three weeklong recesses—a December Holiday Recess, a February Mid-Winter Recess, and Spring Break in April.

Because a certain number of hours of professional development are required for teachers and staff, several half-days appear on the calendar. The first Fridays in February, March, and April are all half-days for students. Teachers and staff spend the rest of those days in workshops.

December is a month of music in the district. There are two high-school concerts, two middle-school concerts, and two elementary-school concerts. Pity the parents with children at each level! Those parents could easily attend two to three concerts a week during that short month.

Special occasions are marked on the calendar. These include visits from scientists and musicians, who come on Wednesdays to lecture or to perform in the auditorium. They also include town functions that might call for student attendance, such as the Dryden Tree Lighting in early December, which often features a chorus of elementary students.

Dates critical for high-school students appear on the calendar, too. Examples include the registration dates for the SAT and ACT exams, dates for Academic Awards presentations, and of course Graduation Day.

Parents and other citizens appreciate the calendar for its inclusion of PTA meeting dates as well as dates and locations of Board of Education meetings and budget presentations. All in all, the annual school calendar is a useful tool for students, faculty, staff, parents, and residents of the town. Most people agree that the small cost of printing and disseminating the school calendar is money well spent.

GO ON TO THE NEXT PAGE

The next seven questions are based on this passage.

6. Which of the following inferences may logically be drawn from the first paragraph of the passage?

   A) There are only three weeks off during the school year.
   B) Students do not get a week off at Thanksgiving time.
   C) All students in Dryden play sports or musical instruments.
   D) Spring Break is the longest of the school holidays.

7. In the third paragraph, which sentence expresses the author's opinion?

   A) The first sentence
   B) The second sentence
   C) The third sentence
   D) The fourth sentence

8. Which paragraph of the passage best represents persuasive writing?

   A) The first paragraph
   B) The second paragraph
   C) The fourth paragraph
   D) The last paragraph

9. Which of the following sentences represents a summary sentence for the passage?

   A) There are three weeklong recesses—a December Holiday Recess, a February Mid-Winter Recess, and Spring Break in April.
   B) Because a certain number of hours of professional development are required for teachers and staff, several half-days appear on the calendar.
   C) Examples include the registration dates for the SAT and ACT exams, dates for Academic Awards presentations, and of course Graduation Day.
   D) All in all, the annual school calendar is a useful tool for students, faculty, staff, parents, and residents of the town.

10. Based on the fourth paragraph, which event might find its way onto the school calendar?

   A) A meeting of the Senior Citizen Council to discuss budget cuts to Medicare
   B) A Rotary Dinner that features scholarship presentations for high school juniors
   C) The annual Arbor Day tree planting by the mayor
   D) Opening day for the State Fair in late August

GO ON TO THE NEXT PAGE

11. Does the title of the passage reflect its theme, topic, main idea, or supporting detail?

   A) Theme
   B) Topic
   C) Main idea
   D) Supporting detail

12. What was the author's purpose in writing this passage?

   A) To explain the features and functions of the school calendar
   B) To compare and contrast various times in the school year
   C) To encourage readers to purchase a school calendar
   D) To tell step-by-step how to use the Dryden school calendar

A sultan was dissatisfied with the quality of his treasure and wished to augment it. He called on several wise men from the kingdom to meet at a certain time in his council room.

The next two questions are based on this passage.

13. Based on the passage, which of the following is a logical prediction of what the sultan will do?

   A) Take the wise men's treasure.
   B) Give his treasure away.
   C) Ask the wise men for ideas.
   D) Send the wise men abroad.

14. Based on a prior knowledge of literature, the reader can infer that this passage was taken from which of the following?

   A) A magazine article
   B) A folktale
   C) A persuasive essay
   D) A language textbook

15. The driver of a rental car wishes to know the location of the car's gas cap release. Which of the following is the most appropriate source of information for that driver?

   A) A website on foreign cars
   B) *Car & Driver* magazine
   C) A road map
   D) The owner's manual

GO ON TO THE NEXT PAGE

16. Read and follow the directions below.

    1. Walk one block east and turn right.

    2. Walk two blocks south and turn left.

    3. Walk two blocks east to your destination.

Where is your destination compared to your original location?

A) 2 blocks east, 2 blocks south
B) 3 blocks east, 3 blocks south
C) 2 blocks east, 3 blocks south
D) 3 blocks east, 2 blocks south

17.

> GED TEST DATES for the year 2016
>
> (This is a two-part test; all dates Friday night and Saturday morning)
>
> April 8 & 9 in Teeburg
>
> May 13 & 14 in Starville
>
> June 3 & 4 in Teeburg
>
> July 10 & 11 in Starville
>
> August 19 & 20 in Teeburg
>
> September 16 & 17 in Starville
>
> Call our office for further details: 555-2929. Final deadline for application is the Friday one week prior to the test. Application forms are available at the Center for New Careers. Apply early—waiting for the deadline may result in losing a seat at the test if we are overbooked.

If you wish to apply to take the third GED test offered in Teeburg, what is the last possible date to hand in your application form?

A) May 27
B) July 3
C) August 12
D) August 19

18. If the jury <u>absolves</u> him, my uncle may be back at work in no time.

Which of the following is the definition of the word *absolves*?

A) Deciphers
B) Clears
C) Settles
D) Includes

GO ON TO THE NEXT PAGE

KITCHEN DESIGN & REMODELING

CK Construction 2 Divan St 555-3910

Foster Custom Kitchens

    24 State St 555-6789

Willet Kitchen & Bath 129 Bly Pl . . . 555-6822

KITCHEN EQUIPMENT

Cookout Landreau Mall 555-2566

Miko Bar & Kitchen 32 State St 555-1700

Sanduhra Foods 421 Burr St 555-0909

KUNG FU INSTRUCTION

See Martial Arts Instruction

LABORATORIES—CLINICAL

Asthma & Allergy Assoc.
    Durham Pl 555-2770

Kiowa Medical Center State St . . . 555-4300

Landreau Mall 555-4311

FOSTER CUSTOM KITCHENS
The finest in cabinetry for over
50 years!

LABORATORIES—DENTAL
Asok Dental 495 Marco Blvd 555-2780
Canto Family Dentistry 422 Burr St . . . 555-8998
Small Dental Lab 877 Fortuna St 555-0065

LABORATORIES—TESTING
Enviro Control 8712 Rte 14 555-8909
Kiowa Medical Center State St 555-4300
Microvac 225 University Pl 555-1330

CANTO FAMILY DENTISTRY
On-site lab for same-day service!
Full-service dentistry for the whole
family: 555-8998

The next two questions are based on this sample yellow page.

19. A customer wonders whether the blender she wants to buy is available in town. Which of the following businesses should she call?

  A) Willet Kitchen & Bath
  B) Foster Custom Kitchens
  C) Miko Bar & Kitchen
  D) Microvac

20. A patient hopes to get a set of x-rays and new dentures all in one day. Which number should she probably call first?

  A) 555-2780
  B) 555-8998
  C) 555-0065
  D) 555-4300

GO ON TO THE NEXT PAGE

21.

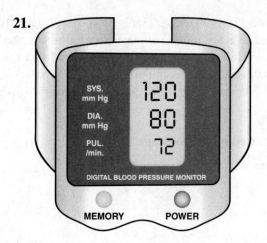

Based on the blood pressure monitor above, what is this patient's pulse rate?

A) 72

B) 80

C) 120

D) $\dfrac{120}{80}$

Weekly Earnings	$560.40
Federal Income Tax	$64.63
State Income Tax	$27.67
FICA (Social Security, Medicaid)	$39.08

22. Penelope receives a statement like this with every weekly paycheck. About how much of her weekly paycheck goes toward income tax?

A) Between 0% and 5%

B) Between 5% and 10%

C) Between 15% and 20%

D) Between 30% and 40%

GO ON TO THE NEXT PAGE

Saturated Fat—A fat that is solid at room temperature and comes <u>principally</u> from animal food products and selected plants. Some examples of saturated fat include foods such as beef, lamb, pork, lard, butter, cream, whole milk, and high-fat cheese. Plant sources include coconut oil, cocoa butter, palm oil, and palm kernel oil. Saturated fat causes high LDL cholesterol levels—a risk for cardiovascular disease.

The next two questions are based on this passage.

23. What does *principally* mean here?

   A) Mostly
   B) First
   C) In our opinion
   D) Royally

24. In this context, what are "selected plants"?

   A) Plants that have been chosen
   B) Particular plants
   C) Top-quality plants
   D) Restricted plants

Abebe Bikila, arguably the world's greatest marathoner, ran barefoot. That should have been a sign to all of us that running barefoot is not only natural but also desirable. As running shoes have gotten lighter and lighter, they have given us the impression that we're going barefoot. However, today's "glove" shoes are even closer to that sensation. Running in these shoes is the best of both worlds. You are protected from pebbles and prickers, but your toes can move, and your feet feel the earth below them.

The next two questions are based on this passage.

25. What is the author's apparent purpose for writing this paragraph about running barefoot?

   A) To explain how to do it
   B) To introduce a great runner
   C) To present an opinion
   D) To entertain the reader

26. In the context of the passage, does the phrase "running in these shoes is the best of both worlds" constitute a topic, a main idea, a theme, or supporting details?

   A) Topic
   B) Main idea
   C) Theme
   D) Supporting details

GO ON TO THE NEXT PAGE

27. A resident of the city wants to alert a reporter to a broken water main in his neighborhood. Which department of the newspaper should he contact?

A) Editorial
B) Business
C) Local news
D) Classified

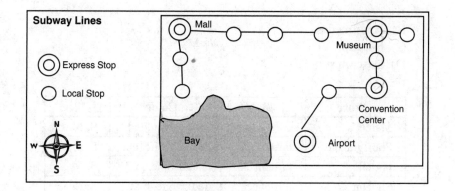

The next two questions are based on this map.

28. A passenger starts at the airport and takes the local subway to the convention center. How many stops is that?

A) 1
B) 2
C) 3
D) 4

29. A passenger boards the local line one stop south of the mall. If she switches to the express line at the first possible chance, how many local stops will she avoid on her way to the museum?

A) 1
B) 2
C) 3
D) 4

GO ON TO THE NEXT PAGE

30. Chapter 3: Early Mathematicians

    A. Zeno
    B. Archimedes
    C. Einstein
    D. Descartes

Analyze the headings above. Which of the following headings is out of place?

A) Zeno
B) Archimedes
C) Einstein
D) Descartes

31.

Store	Style	Color	Size
Marcel's	crew neck	blue, green, red	S, M, L
Pomegranate	turtleneck	black, white, tan	S, M, L
Fortelli	turtleneck	black, blue, gray	S, M
Simeon's	turtleneck	red, white, blue	S, L

A customer wants to buy a blue turtleneck in size medium. Which store's supply will suit her best?

A) Marcel's
B) Pomegranate
C) Fortelli
D) Simeon's

32. A high school junior wants to improve his score on the SATs. Which of the following is an appropriate resource for that student?

A) An encyclopedia
B) A study guide
C) A grammar book
D) A teacher's manual

GO ON TO THE NEXT PAGE

33. Memory, 249–251

In the book whose index is excerpted above, which pages probably contain the chapter on human reproduction?

A) 230–239
B) 240–252
C) 253–275
D) 276–290

34. Start with this shape. Follow the directions to alter its appearance.

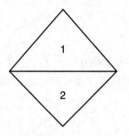

1. Rotate the entire shape 90 degrees to the right.
2. Remove section 1 from the shape.
3. Draw a circle that encloses the new shape.

Which of the following represents the shape after these alterations?

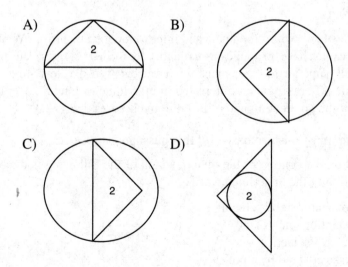

A)   B)

C)   D)

GO ON TO THE NEXT PAGE

35. After resting briefly at mile 12, the marathoner continued with a somewhat more uneven gait.

Which word from the sentence above has a negative connotation?

A) resting
B) briefly
C) somewhat
D) uneven

36. Chapter 4: Civil War

    1. Key Battles

        A. Antietam
        B. Bull Run
        C. Chancellorsville
        D. _____
        E. Manassas Gap

Examine the headings above. Based on what you see, which of the following is a reasonable heading to insert in the blank spot?

A) Waterloo
B) Thermopylae
C) Vicksburg
D) Bunker Hill

This memo was sent to employees from the director of human resources.

To: All Staff

From: Helen Jameson, HR

Re: Dental Plan

Beginning July 1, we will offer a new and improved dental plan from Whitby Insurance. We must have 30 applicants to qualify for the lowest rates. This plan is substantially superior to other plans we have reviewed. Packets are available in the HR office. If you are interested in individual or family <u>coverage</u>, please fill out the application and return it to me before June 1.

The next two questions are based on this passage.

37. Based on the context of the memo, which of the following is the best definition of the underlined word?

A) Concealment by screening
B) Extent of a news story
C) Defensive tactics
D) Risks covered by a policy

GO ON TO THE NEXT PAGE

38. Which of the following statements best describes Ms. Jameson's biases?

A) She has no bias about the dental plan.
B) She has a bias in favor of the new plan.
C) She has a bias in opposition to the new plan.
D) Her biases are hidden and impossible to assess.

Adder's Tongue or Serpent's Tongue

from *Complete Herbal* by Nicholas Culpeper

Descript: This herb has but one leaf, which grows with the stalk a finger's length above the ground, being flat and of a fresh green colour; broad like Water Plantain, but less, without any rib in it; from the bottom of which leaf, on the inside, rises up (ordinarily) one, sometimes two or three slender stalks, the upper half whereof is somewhat bigger, and dented with small dents of a yellowish green colour, like the tongue of an adder serpent (only this is as useful as they are formidable). The roots continue all the year.

Place: It grows in moist meadows, and such like places.

Time: It is to be found in May or April, for it quickly perishes with a little heat.

Government and virtues: It is an herb under the dominion of the Moon and Cancer, and therefore if the weakness of the retentive faculty be caused by an evil influence of Saturn in any part of the body governed by the Moon, or under the dominion of Cancer, this herb cures it by sympathy. It cures these diseases after specified, in any part of the body under the influence of Saturn, by antipathy.

The next two questions are based on this passage.

39. The author's comparison of Serpent's Tongue to Water Plantain is an example of which of the following?

A) Topic
B) Main idea
C) Theme
D) Supporting details

40. Which of the following statements best reflects the author's culturally held beliefs about herbal medicine?

A) It is not as effective or useful as Western medicine.
B) Its effectiveness is influenced by astrological events.
C) It should be used in tandem with traditional methods.
D) Its use should be controlled by expert practitioners.

GO ON TO THE NEXT PAGE

41. Read and follow the directions below.

   1. Imagine a measuring cup that holds 16 ounces.
   2. Fill the cup halfway with water.
   3. Pour out 4 ounces.
   4. Add back 6 ounces.
   5. Pour out 1 ounce.

How many ounces of water are now in the cup?

   A) 8 ounces
   B) 9 ounces
   C) 10 ounces
   D) 11 ounces

42. A student reading a history book about World War II wishes to find the book's first reference to General Patton. Where should the student look?

   A) In the index
   B) In the table of contents
   C) In the preface
   D) In the glossary

43.

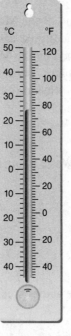

On the thermometer above, what is the current temperature in degrees Celsius?

   A) 24°
   B) 28°
   C) 76°
   D) 80°

GO ON TO THE NEXT PAGE

Nutrition Facts

Serving size 2 tbsp (32 g)
Servings per container 16

Amount per serving

Calories 10	Calories from fat 0

	% Daily value*
Total fat 0 g	0%
Saturated fat 0 g	0%
Trans fat 0 g	
Cholesterol 0 mg	0%
Sodium 95 mg	4%
Total carbohydrate 2 g	1%
Dietary fiber 1 g	4%
Sugars 1 g	
Protein 0 g	

Vitamin A 6%	•	Vitamin C 10%
Calcium 0%	•	Iron 0%

• Percent daily values are based on a 2,000 calorie diet. Your daily values may be higher or lower depending on your calorie needs:

The next two questions are based on this chart.

44. A consumer eats one serving of this product. How much of his daily vitamin C intake does he have yet to consume?

   A) 10%
   B) 14%
   C) 84%
   D) 90%

45. Diane is on a diet of 1,500 calories a day. When it comes to Diane's diet, what is true of the sodium value of one serving of the product above?

   A) The daily value in Diane's diet is greater than 4 percent.
   B) The daily value in Diane's diet is less than 4 percent.
   C) The daily value in Diane's diet is equal to 4 percent.
   D) The answer cannot be determined from the information given.

GO ON TO THE NEXT PAGE

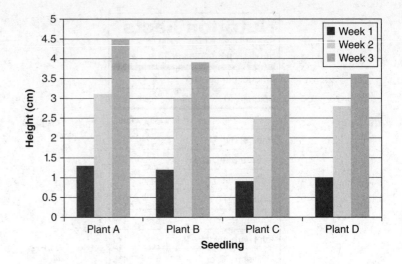

The next two questions are based on this graph.

46. Which plant was tallest after week 1?

A) Plant A
B) Plant B
C) Plant C
D) Plant D

47. Which statement is true?

A) The greatest growth for each plant came in week 1.
B) The greatest growth for each plant came in week 2.
C) The greatest growth for each plant came in week 3.
D) Two plants had greater growth in week 3 than in week 2.

48. Before pouring the liquid into the <u>mold</u>, the artist made sure that the temperature was exactly right.

Based on the context of the sentence above, which of the following is the definition of the underlined word?

A) Fashion
B) Cast
C) Fungus
D) Character

GO ON TO THE NEXT PAGE

Making Voting Mandatory

In some nations, voting is compulsory, and those who do not go to the polls are fined. If voting is a duty, why shouldn't it be mandatory? We make other civic duties mandatory, among them paying taxes, going to school, registering for the draft, and serving on a jury.

If voting were mandatory in the United States, we would be assured that every elected candidate truly represented the will of the majority. It would be far more difficult for special interests to influence elections if all adults 18 and older actually voted. In addition, it would be impossible to impose restrictions on the right to vote.

The next two questions are based on this passage.

49. Which of the following statements would best support the writer's argument?

    A) Some American citizens have no interest in voting.
    B) In our country, voting is actually a right, not a duty.
    C) The role of money in politics may decrease if everyone votes.
    D) It is possible to vote without knowing anything about the issues.

50. Which of the following conclusions is best supported by the passage?

    A) Mandatory voting will never happen until citizens express their desire to make it happen.
    B) Mandatory voting could make the system fairer and more representative.
    C) Mandatory voting works best in nations where there are few obstacles to voting.
    D) Mandatory voting would be difficult to impose on our disparate, diverse electorate.

51. Dr. Morgan dropped the beaker; _____, the room was closed for six hours until it could be properly detoxified.

Which word or phrase would best complete the sentence?

    A) however
    B) likewise
    C) as a result
    D) meanwhile

GO ON TO THE NEXT PAGE

52. Which of these statements about polio is a fact?

A) The polio virus was identified in 1908 by Karl Landsteiner.
B) We should be glad that polio has been nearly eradicated.
C) The outbreak of polio in 20th-century Europe was terrifying.
D) Polio has distressing effects, which may include paralysis.

53. Was the *casus belli* of World War I really the assassination of the archduke?

How are italics used in the sentence?

A) To stress important words
B) To signify words in another language
C) To identify the title of a work
D) To delineate a scientific term

STOP. THIS IS THE END OF PART I.

Part II. Mathematics

36 items (32 scored), 54 minutes

1. Express $\frac{2}{5}$ as a decimal.

   A) 0.2
   B) 0.25
   C) 0.4
   D) 2.5

2. Early Bird Café sold 24 café frappes between 6 and 7 A.M., 30 between 7 and 8 A.M., 45 between 8 and 9 A.M., and 17 between 9 and 10 A.M. What was the café's average sale of café frappes over that 4-hour period?

   A) 28
   B) 29
   C) 32
   D) 37.5

3. Tamison bought twenty 29-cent stamps and forty 42-cent stamps. If she gave the postal worker $25, how much change did she receive?

   A) $2.40
   B) $2.80
   C) $3.20
   D) $3.60

4. What is the product of the numbers 0.15×0.52?

   A) 0.0078
   B) 0.078
   C) 0.78
   D) 7.8

5. How many feet are in 6 meters? (Note: 1 meter = 3.28 feet.)

   A) 1.83 feet
   B) 18.48 feet
   C) 18.8 feet
   D) 19.68 feet

6. If a helicopter flies at about 80 mph, how long will it take to travel 140 miles?

   A) 1 hour 15 minutes
   B) 1 hour 20 minutes
   C) 1 hour 30 minutes
   D) 1 hour 45 minutes

GO ON TO THE NEXT PAGE

7. Donald earns 8% of the selling price of each house he sells. If he sells a house for $152,000, how much does he earn?

A) $12,160
B) $14,040
C) $19,000
D) $21,600

8. $(x + 3)(x + 3)$

Simplify the expression above. Which of the following is correct?

A) $x^2 + 6x + 6$
B) $x^2 + 6x + 9$
C) $2x^2 + 6x + 9$
D) $2x^2 + 9x + 9$

9. What is the approximate circumference of a circle with a radius of 3 centimeters?

A) 9 cm
B) 19 cm
C) 28 cm
D) 42 cm

10.

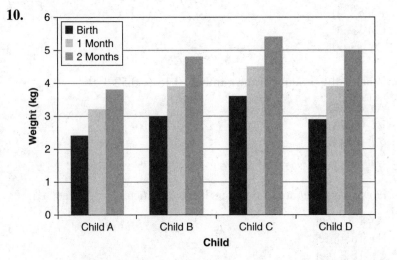

The graph above shows the weight gain over time of four newborns.

Which child showed the greatest weight gain between birth and 2 months?

A) Child A
B) Child B
C) Child C
D) Child D

GO ON TO THE NEXT PAGE

11.

Albany				
284	Buffalo			
153	370	Flushing		
219	75	325	Rochester	
135	152	261	87	Syracuse

This mileage chart shows the distances in miles between certain New York cities.

How much farther is it from Buffalo to Flushing than from Buffalo to Syracuse?

A) 283 miles
B) 218 miles
C) 128 miles
D) 45 miles

12. $\dfrac{2}{15} + \dfrac{1}{12}$

Simplify the expression above. Which of the following is correct?

A) $\dfrac{1}{9}$

B) $\dfrac{13}{60}$

C) $\dfrac{7}{15}$

D) $\dfrac{11}{12}$

13. Annual salaries at ABC Company range from $23,000 to $106,000. If the median of the salaries is $55,000, and there are 20 employees, what must be true?

A) The median of the salaries is less than the average.
B) At least two workers make $23,000 a year.
C) More workers make $106,000 than make $23,000.
D) Ten workers make $55,000 or less, and ten make $55,000 or more.

14. What is the product of 2.4 × 4.2?

A) 1.008
B) 10.08
C) 10.8
D) 18

GO ON TO THE NEXT PAGE

15. How many liters are there in 2,500 milliliters?

A) 2.5 liters
B) 25 liters
C) 250 liters
D) 25,000,000 liters

16.

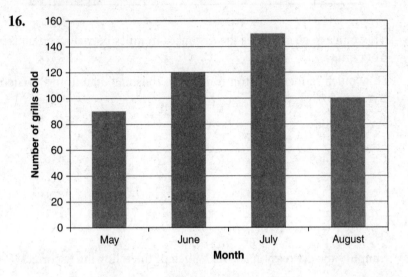

The graph above shows the number of grills sold by one outdoors store over the course of 4 months.

During the summer months (June–August), sales of grills amounted to

A) 150 units sold.
B) 270 units sold.
C) 370 units sold.
D) 460 units sold.

17.

Age	Nighttime	Matinee
under 12	$6.50	$4.50
12–64	$8.00	$6.50
65 and over	$7.00	$5.50

This table shows ticket prices at a movie theater.

How much in all would a group of 20 over-65 patrons from the Retired Teachers Club save by attending a matinee rather than a nighttime movie?

A) $20.00
B) $25.00
C) $30.00
D) $35.00

GO ON TO THE NEXT PAGE

18. $5\dfrac{1}{4} - 3\dfrac{5}{6}$

Simplify the expression above. Which of the following is correct?

A) $2\dfrac{1}{6}$

B) $1\dfrac{1}{2}$

C) $1\dfrac{7}{24}$

D) $1\dfrac{5}{12}$

19. $4 \times 3 + (3 + 5) - 6$

Simplify the expression above. Which of the following is correct?

A) 14
B) 13
C) 12
D) 11

20. As boys age, their voices deepen.

Which is the dependent variable in the statement above?

A) Gender
B) Deepness of voice
C) Age of boys
D) Number of boys

21. Which of the following decimal numbers is approximately equal to $\sqrt{18}$?

A) 3.5
B) 3.95
C) 4.2
D) 4.25

22. Professor Quarto ordered 20 laptops for his computer lab at a cost of $895 apiece. Which of the following is an accurate estimate of the cost of the laptops?

A) $16,000
B) $17,000
C) $18,000
D) $19,000

GO ON TO THE NEXT PAGE

23. $4\dfrac{5}{8} \div 1\dfrac{1}{2}$

Simplify the expression above. Which of the following is correct?

A) $4\dfrac{1}{24}$

B) $3\dfrac{23}{24}$

C) $3\dfrac{1}{12}$

D) $3\dfrac{1}{16}$

24.

First hour	$3
Each 30 minutes after first hour	$1
24-hour discount rate	$30

This table shows the parking rates for the central terminal area at an airport.

George parked at the lot for $2\dfrac{1}{2}$ hours. How much did he owe?

A) $5.00
B) $6.00
C) $7.00
D) $7.50

25. At the Farmer's Market, James bought 6 lemons for $1.44. How many lemons did Casey buy for $4.80?

A) 12
B) 18
C) 20
D) 24

26. $(x + 5)(x + 1)$

Simplify the expression above. Which of the following is correct?

A) $x^2 + 6$
B) $x^2 + 6x + 5$
C) $x^2 + 6x + 6$
D) $2x^2 + 6x + 5$

GO ON TO THE NEXT PAGE

27. 75% of what number is 18?

   A) 15
   B) 24
   C) 30
   D) 80

28. In a scale drawing for a toy rocket, 1 inch = 6 inches. If a rocket is 6 inches tall on the drawing, how tall will it be in reality?

   A) 1 foot
   B) 6 feet
   C) 1 yard
   D) 2 yards

29. A scientist must measure the distance between two twigs in a nest. Which would be the most accurate tool to use for this task?

   A) Meter stick
   B) Tape measure
   C) Ruler
   D) Caliper

30. $|5| + |-3|$

   Simplify the expression above.

   A) 2
   B) 3
   C) 5
   D) 8

31. A number is four more than half a given number.

   Translate this phrase into a mathematical expression.

   A) $\dfrac{(n + 4)}{2}$
   B) $n + 2$
   C) $\dfrac{n}{2} - 4$
   D) $\dfrac{n}{2} + 4$

GO ON TO THE NEXT PAGE

32. Order this list of numbers from least to greatest.

$$\sqrt{9}, \frac{14}{4}, 3.14, 3\%$$

A) $\sqrt{9}, 3.14, 3\%, \frac{14}{4}$

B) $3\%, \sqrt{9}, 3.14, \frac{14}{4}$

C) $3\%, \sqrt{9}, \frac{14}{4}, 3.14$

D) $\sqrt{9}, 3\%, 3.14, \frac{14}{4}$

33. Which type of graph would best demonstrate a temperature pattern over the course of several weeks?

A) Line graph
B) Histogram
C) Circle graph
D) Scatter plot

34. Olivia wants to earn $4,500 over the summer to help with college expenses. She earns $15 per hour in a day-care center and $18 per hour as a lifeguard. She is guaranteed 125 hours of lifeguarding time in July and August. How many hours will she need to spend at the day-care center to reach her goal?

A) 75
B) 100
C) 120
D) 150

GO ON TO THE NEXT PAGE

35.

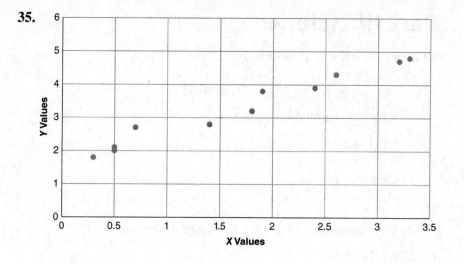

What can you conclude about the relationship between x and y on the graph above?

A) As x increases, y decreases.
B) As x decreases, y increases.
C) As x increases, y increases.
D) No relationship exists.

36. Janelle bought 1 adult ticket and 3 student tickets for the show.

Which of the following algebraic expressions represents what she paid?

A) $x + 3x$
B) $x + 3y$
C) $4x$
D) $x + y$

STOP. THIS IS THE END OF PART II.

Part III. Science

53 items (47 scored), 63 minutes

1. The esophagus is _____ to the stomach.

   Which of the following correctly completes the sentence above?

   A) posterior
   B) lateral
   C) proximal
   D) superior

2. Which would be an anterior feature of the human head?

   A) The nose
   B) The ears
   C) The occipital lobe
   D) The temporal lobe

3. While conducting an experiment, a scientist determines that the data do not support the original theory. This determination corresponds to which of the following steps in the scientific method?

   A) Formulating a hypothesis
   B) Collecting data
   C) Analyzing data
   D) Drawing a conclusion

4. The arteries are part of the _____ system.

   Which of the following correctly completes the sentence above?

   A) nervous
   B) endocrine
   C) lymphatic
   D) cardiovascular

5. Nearly all the gaseous exchanges between air and blood take place at the level of the

   A) pleura.
   B) trachea.
   C) bronchioles.
   D) alveoli.

GO ON TO THE NEXT PAGE

6. How do the intercostal muscles between the ribs assist with respiration?

   A) By protecting the delicate bronchioles and alveoli
   B) By signaling a decrease in intraalveolar pressure
   C) By enlarging and reducing the space in the thorax
   D) By maintaining a medial separation between pleurae

7. What do micrometers, chronometers, and phonometers have in common.

   A) All are measurement tools.
   B) All involve timing of experiments.
   C) All describe distances.
   D) All are related to qualitative data.

8.

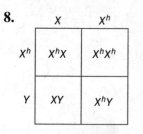

Hemophilia is a sex-linked trait. In the example above of a male with hemophilia and a female carrier, what ratio of the offspring are predicted to have the disease?

   A) 0 female : 2 male
   B) 1 female : 1 male
   C) 1 female : 2 male
   D) 2 female : 1 male

GO ON TO THE NEXT PAGE

9.

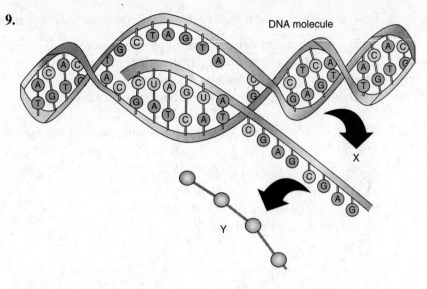

In the diagram above, what process is illustrated by X?

A) Transcription
B) Translation
C) Replication
D) Coding

10.

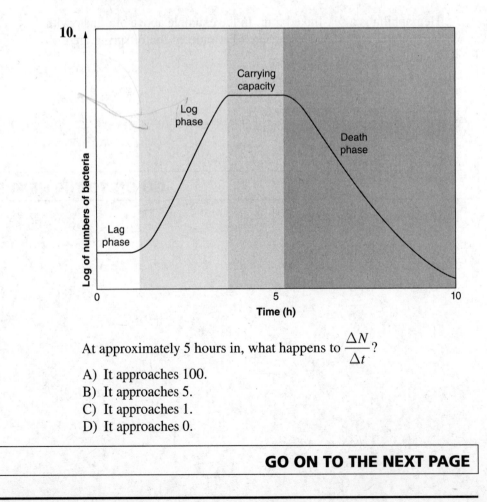

At approximately 5 hours in, what happens to $\dfrac{\Delta N}{\Delta t}$?

A) It approaches 100.
B) It approaches 5.
C) It approaches 1.
D) It approaches 0.

GO ON TO THE NEXT PAGE

11. How should a researcher test the hypothesis that eating chocolate leads to acne in teenagers?

A) Take 100 teenagers and feed each one a different amount of chocolate daily for 60 days; then test for acne.

B) Take 100 teenagers and feed 50 two bars of chocolate daily for 60 days while the other 50 eat no chocolate; then test for acne.

C) Take 1 teenager and feed him or her two bars of chocolate for 30 days and no chocolate for 30 days; then test for acne.

D) Take 100 teenagers and feed them no chocolate for 30 days and two bars of chocolate apiece for 30 days; then test for acne.

12. To determine whether pollution lessened with the depth of a lake, divers collected samples at depths of 1, 2, 3, and 4 meters. After a visual inspection, samples were tested for turbidity and for levels of two pollutants—nitrates and ammonia. Although turbidity increased with depth, amounts of pollutants remained constant.

What would be a logical next step for the researchers?

A) Continue to test at lower depths.

B) Perform the same test in saltwater.

C) Repeat the visual inspection after 12 hours.

D) Repeat the collection and testing of samples 1 week later.

GO ON TO THE NEXT PAGE

13.

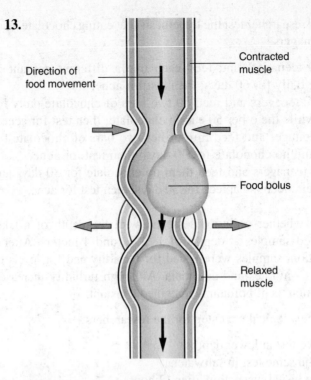

Direction of
food movement

Contracted
muscle

Food bolus

Relaxed
muscle

What does this diagram show?

A) Homeostasis
B) Peristalsis
C) Oxidation
D) Epithelial transport

14. Vitamin D may be replenished through fortified milk and

A) sunshine.
B) protein.
C) fluoride.
D) exercise.

15. Lack of vitamin C may lead to the condition known as

A) kwashiorkor.
B) pellagra.
C) rickets.
D) scurvy.

GO ON TO THE NEXT PAGE

16. A kilogram of air is compressed from 1 m³ to 0.5 m³. Which statement is true?

A) The density is doubled.
B) The density is halved.
C) The mass is doubled.
D) The mass is halved.

17. You contain two odorous gases in vials with porous plugs. Gas A has twice the mass of gas B. Which observation is most likely?

A) You will smell gas A before you smell gas B.
B) You will smell gas B before you smell gas A.
C) You will smell gas A but not gas B.
D) You will smell gas B but not gas A.

18. Which of the following parts of the brain has the most to do with memory?

A) Basal ganglia
B) Cerebellum
C) Hippocampus
D) Medulla oblongata

19. Which is the first step in urine production?

A) Passage of fluid through the peritubular capillaries
B) Filtration of blood through the glomerulus
C) Secretion of solutes into the nephron
D) Reabsorption of water in the Loop of Henle

20. Which of the following is an example of passive immunity?

A) Live (attenuated) vaccine
B) Inactivated vaccine with a booster shot
C) Transfer of antibodies through breast milk
D) T-cells attacking a pathogen in the body

GO ON TO THE NEXT PAGE

21.

PERIODIC TABLE OF THE ELEMENTS

1 H																	2 He
3 Li	4 Be											5 B	6 C	7 N	8 O	9 F	10 Ne
11 Na	12 Mg											13 Al	14 Si	15 P	16 S	17 Ci	18 Ar
19 K	20 Ca	21 Sc	22 Ti	23 V	24 Cr	25 Mn	26 Fe	27 Co	28 Ni	29 Cu	30 Zn	31 Ga	32 Ge	33 As	34 Se	35 Br	36 Kr
37 Rb	38 Sr	39 Y	40 Z	41 Nb	42 Mo	43 Tc	44 Ru	45 Rh	46 Pd	47 Ag	48 Cd	49 In	50 Sn	51 Sb	52 Te	53 I	54 Xe
55 Cs	56 Ba	see below	72 Hf	73 Ta	74 W	75 Re	76 Os	77 It	78 Pt	79 Au	80 Hg	81 Ti	82 Pb	83 Bi	84 Po	85 At	86 Rn
87 Fr	88 Ra	see below	104 Rf	105 Db	106 Sg	107 Bh	108 Hs	109 Mt	110 Ds	111 Rg	112 Uub	113 Uut	114 Uuq	115 Uup	116 Uuh	117 Uus	118 Uuo

■ = Alkali Metals   ▒ = Halogens   ░ = Noble Gases

RARE EARTH ELEMENTS

Lanthanides	57 La	58 Ce	59 Pr	60 Nd	61 Pm	62 Sm	63 Eu	64 Gd	65 Tb	66 Dy	67 Ho	68 Er	69 Tm	70 Yb	71 Lu
Actinides	89 Ac	90 Th	91 Pa	92 U	93 Np	94 Pu	95 Am	96 Cm	97 Bk	98 Cf	99 Es	100 Fm	101 Md	102 No	103 Lr

Which pair of elements are most alike in reactivity?

A) He and H
B) K and Ar
C) Cl and P
D) Ba and Mg

GO ON TO THE NEXT PAGE

22.

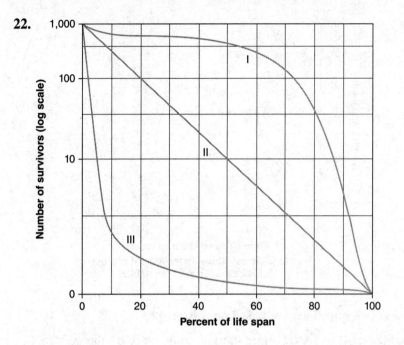

A ground squirrel has a relatively constant death rate. Which survivor-ship curve indicates the life span of a ground squirrel?

A) I
B) II
C) III
D) None of the above

GO ON TO THE NEXT PAGE

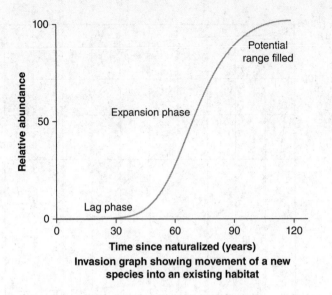

**Invasion graph showing movement of a new
species into an existing habitat**

The next two questions are based on this graph.

23. Suppose this species were introduced in 1960. By the year 2020, you
    would expect to see

    A) the species just beginning to expand.
    B) the species occupying less than a tenth of its potential range.
    C) the species occupying just under half of its potential range.
    D) the species reaching the limits of its distribution.

24. What would be the best time to intervene in an invasion of unwanted
    weeds?

    A) Before the invasion begins
    B) During the lag phase
    C) In the middle of the expansion phase
    D) After the potential range is filled

25. Which kind of protein fiber is *not* found in connective tissue?

    A) Fibrin
    B) Elastic
    C) Collagen
    D) Reticular

GO ON TO THE NEXT PAGE

26.

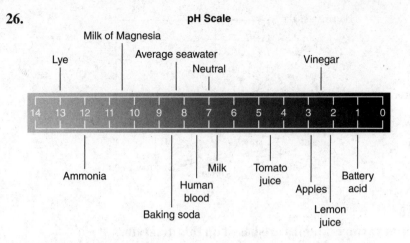

pH Scale

Where would you expect tap water to fall on the scale shown?

A) Between 1 and 3
B) Between 4 and 6
C) Between 6 and 8
D) Between 8 and 10

27. A first-degree burn features damage to which of the following?

A) Epidermis
B) Dermis
C) Epidermis and dermis
D) Epidermis, dermis, and hypodermis

28. What is the main function of the sebaceous gland?

A) Stimulation of the appetite
B) Reduction of body temperature
C) Lubrication of the hair and skin
D) Protection of the tracheal lining

29. Someone who has undergone a splenectomy is likely to be prone to which of the following?

A) Infection
B) Depression
C) Necrosis
D) Intestinal blockage

GO ON TO THE NEXT PAGE

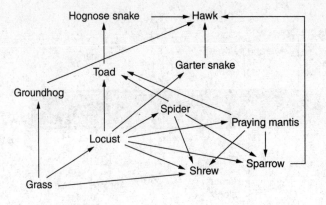

The next two questions are based on this diagram.

30. Which of these animals occupies the highest trophic level?

    A) Toad
    B) Locust
    C) Spider
    D) Hawk

31. When species X was introduced into this system, the number of snakes increased, while the number of shrews decreased. Species X was probably

    A) a plant.
    B) a primary consumer.
    C) a secondary consumer.
    D) a predator.

32. How does the integumentary system work with the nervous system?

    A) The integumentary system removes heat from the neurons in the nervous system.
    B) The nervous system circulates nutrients outward to the integumentary system.
    C) Touch input via the integumentary system sends messages to the nervous system.
    D) Messages from the nervous system affect the color and texture of the skin.

33. The organ system primarily responsible for storing minerals is the _____ system.

    Which of the following correctly completes the sentence above?

    A) skeletal
    B) endocrine
    C) lymphatic
    D) cardiovascular

GO ON TO THE NEXT PAGE

34. Sublimation is the change in matter from solid to gas without passing through a liquid phase. Outside of the laboratory, which solid provides the best example of this?

A) Iron
B) Silver
C) Salt crystal
D) Dry ice

35. A researcher looked for a correlation between students' test scores and the amount of sleep they got the night before the test. The results were as follows.

Score	85	74	69	78	90	88	73
Sleep hrs.	5	8	9	6	6	8	9

How would you describe the correlation between scores and hours of sleep?

A) Direct
B) Inverse
C) No correlation
D) Logarithmic

36. In an experiment designed to contrast flu infection rates in kindergarteners in urban and rural schools, which variable might be considered extraneous?

A) Age
B) Illness
C) Gender
D) Habitat

37. Which structure is part of the upper respiratory tract?

A) Laryngopharynx
B) Left main bronchus
C) Trachea
D) Thoracic diaphragm

38. Which disease is most likely to result in height loss?

A) Osteoporosis
B) Scleroderma
C) Celiac disease
D) Hepatitis A

GO ON TO THE NEXT PAGE

39. Which gland is located superior to the kidney?

A) Pituitary
B) Adrenal
C) Hypothalamus
D) Pancreas

40. What results from the second stage of meiosis?

A) Two haploid cells
B) Four haploid cells
C) Two diploid cells
D) Four diploid cells

41. The weak bonds between bases in a double helix always include an atom of _____.

Which of the following correctly completes the sentence above?

A) helium
B) carbon
C) hydrogen
D) phosphorus

42. Which body part is *not* involved in the production of semen?

A) Seminal vesicle
B) Prostate gland
C) Testicles
D) Urethra

43. Bears, starfish, and toads belong to the same

A) species.
B) phylum.
C) family.
D) kingdom.

44. Which of the following is a main function of the lymph nodes?

A) Absorbing
B) Filtering
C) Regulating
D) Fusing

GO ON TO THE NEXT PAGE

45. Where does the conversion of ammonia to urea take place?

    A) In the liver
    B) In the large intestine
    C) In the kidneys
    D) In the gallbladder

46. What type of muscle tissue is contained in the walls of the body's hollow organs?

    A) Smooth
    B) Striated
    C) Cardiac
    D) Skeletal

47. Which T cells stimulate the production of antibodies by B cells?

    A) Suppressor T cells
    B) Helper T cells
    C) Cytotoxic T cells
    D) Both A and B

48. What prevents food from entering the windpipe?

    A) The uvula
    B) The trachea
    C) The epiglottis
    D) Peristalsis

49. Into which chamber of the heart does deoxygenated blood first flow?

    A) Left atrium
    B) Right atrium
    C) Left ventricle
    D) Right ventricle

50. The digestion of which product begins with the secretion of salivary amylase?

    A) Protein
    B) Lipid
    C) Starch
    D) Amino acid

51. Which part of the nervous system is termed involuntary?

    A) Somatic
    B) Autonomic
    C) Central
    D) Peripheral

GO ON TO THE NEXT PAGE

52. Which hormone stimulates uterine contractions?

    A) Oxytocin

    B) Progesterone

    C) Estrogen

    D) Prednisone

53. Overpopulation occurs when the _____ in a region exceeds the _____.

Which of the following correctly completes the sentence above?

    A) crude birth rate; crude death rate

    B) crude death rate; crude birth rate

    C) infant mortality rate; morbidity rate

    D) morbidity rate; infant mortality rate

STOP. THIS IS THE END OF PART III.

Part IV. English and Language Usage

28 items (24 scored), 28 minutes

1. Shaka _____ completed her residency.

   Which of the following correctly completes the sentence above?

   A) finaly
   B) finally
   C) finely
   D) final

2. The puppy chased _____ tail as the children watched _____.

   Which of the following correctly completes the sentence above?

   A) its; delightedly
   B) it's; delightedly
   C) its; delitedly
   D) it's; delitedly

3. Three days from now, the horses _____.

   Which of the following correctly completes the sentence above?

   A) performing in a show
   B) performed in a show
   C) will perform in a show
   D) have performed in a show

4. The iterate teacher moved continually from one school to another within the district.

   What is the error in this sentence?

   A) iterate
   B) continually
   C) within
   D) district

5. Too many potential job choices put Martin in a quandary.

   What is the simple predicate of this sentence?

   A) potential
   B) choices
   C) put
   D) Martin

GO ON TO THE NEXT PAGE

6. The magician's adroitness and masterful skill both surprised and elated his audience of young people.

Which words are redundant in the sentence above?

A) adroitness, masterful
B) adroitness, skill
C) surprised, elated
D) audience, young people

7. The substance of his speech on income inequality fascinated us.

What is the meaning of *substance* in the sentence above?

A) Dependable quality
B) Physical matter
C) Subject matter
D) Wealth and possessions

8. Which of these sentences represents the conclusion of a paragraph?

A) Olivia's internship in Baltimore was a fascinating experience.
B) Not only did she learn a trade, but she also learned life skills.
C) She worked for a construction firm that was building a hotel.
D) She lived in a tiny apartment and cooked for herself each night.

9. Every so often the friends get together to dish and enjoy a quick meal.

Which word in the sentence above is slang?

A) so often
B) get
C) dish
D) meal

10. Which sentence is the clearest?

A) At the age of seven, my mother moved me to a new school.
B) When I was seven, my mother moved me to a new school.
C) At the age of seven, I moved my mother to a new school.
D) My mother, at the age of seven, moved me to a new school.

GO ON TO THE NEXT PAGE

11. The book is in my locker at school that is long overdue.

Which phrase or clause is misplaced in the sentence above?

A) The book
B) in my locker
C) at school
D) that is long overdue

12. Which of the sentences below is most clear and correct?

A) We quickly consumed the picnic lunch she had made.
B) We consumed the picnic lunch she quickly had made.
C) We consumed the picnic lunch quickly she had made.
D) Quickly the picnic lunch she had made we consumed.

13. The nursing staff _____ to serve their patients well.

Which of the following correctly completes the sentence above?

A) hope
B) hopes
C) hoping
D) does hope

14. Until the semester ends, Lily _____.

Which of the following correctly completes the sentence above?

A) is not traveling far from town
B) has not traveled far from town
C) will not have traveled far from town
D) will not travel far from town

15. The ingenuous foxes managed to lever open one side of the coop.

What is the error in this sentence?

A) ingenuous
B) foxes
C) lever
D) coop

GO ON TO THE NEXT PAGE

16. Endangered baby <u>animals</u> are easy to market as the face of environmental protection; people consider _____ too precious to harm.

Which of the following options correctly completes the sentence? The antecedent of the pronoun to be added is underlined.

A) it
B) him
C) them
D) they

17. The general made the following statement before leading his men into battle _____ "Do your best, and know that I respect your courage."

Which of the following punctuation marks correctly completes the sentence above?

A) ;
B) :
C) -
D) ,

18. Please don't wait _____ long _____ complete the survey.

Which of the following sets of words should be used to fill in the blanks in the sentence above?

A) too; two
B) to; too
C) two; to
D) too; to

19. Stuart hopes that no one will _____ his presentation.

Which of the following is the correct completion of the sentence above?

A) criticize
B) criticice
C) critacize
D) critisize

20. In which word does the suffix change a noun to a verb?

A) Community
B) Hospitalize
C) Teachable
D) Mythology

GO ON TO THE NEXT PAGE

21. Which of the following is an example of a correctly punctuated sentence?

    A) Don't you love their rich sweet scent? asked Mona, holding up a flower.
    B) "Don't you love their rich sweet scent," asked Mona holding up a flower.
    C) "Don't you love their rich, sweet scent?" asked Mona, holding up a flower.
    D) "Don't you love their rich, sweet scent," asked Mona, holding up a flower?

22. During the demonstration, my backpack had been stolen.

    Which of the following changes the sentence above so that it is written in the active rather than in the passive voice?

    A) During the demonstration, someone stole my backpack.
    B) My backpack had been stolen during the demonstration.
    C) My backpack, during the demonstration, had been stolen.
    D) During the demonstration, my backpack was stolen.

23. Which of the following sentences has correct subject-verb agreement?

    A) One of the kittens prefer the dog's food to its own.
    B) Several in that factory supports the local union.
    C) Either of those medications lowers high cholesterol.
    D) Someone in the library stacks sneeze several times.

24. The _____ of the drums delighted the crowd of children.

    Which of the following is the correct completion of the sentence above?

    A) rhythem
    B) rythm
    C) rhythm
    D) rithm

25. The bird's mangled wing would keep it from flying for many months.

    The word *mangled* serves as which of the following parts of speech in the sentence above?

    A) Noun
    B) Pronoun
    C) Verb
    D) Adjective

GO ON TO THE NEXT PAGE

26. Which of the following book titles is correctly capitalized?

A) *The Coast of Maine*
B) *Insider's Guide to The Maine Coast*
C) *Maine's most scenic Roads*
D) *Hidden History Of Maine*

27. Which of the following is an example of a simple sentence?

A) The pharmacy at the corner shut down after the much larger drive-in pharmacy opened nearby.
B) The corner pharmacy had to close due to competition from the much larger drive-in pharmacy.
C) Once a larger, drive-in pharmacy moved into the area, the corner pharmacy folded.
D) The corner pharmacy thrived until a new, larger pharmacy opened.

28. Which of the following is the best definition of the word *antenatal*?

A) Against birth
B) Near water
C) Before birth
D) Underwater

STOP. THIS IS THE END OF TEAS PRACTICE TEST 2.

TEAS Practice Test 2: Answer Key

PART I: READING

1. C	19. C	37. D
2. A	20. B	38. B
3. A	21. A	39. D
4. A	22. C	40. B
5. B	23. A	41. B
6. B	24. B	42. A
7. C	25. C	43. A
8. D	26. B	44. D
9. D	27. C	45. A
10. B	28. B	46. A
11. B	29. C	47. B
12. A	30. C	48. B
13. C	31. C	49. C
14. B	32. B	50. B
15. D	33. D	51. C
16. D	34. B	52. A
17. C	35. D	53. B
18. B	36. C	

PART II: MATHEMATICS

1. C	13. D	25. C
2. B	14. B	26. B
3. A	15. A	27. B
4. B	16. C	28. C
5. D	17. C	29. D
6. D	18. D	30. D
7. A	19. A	31. D
8. B	20. B	32. B
9. B	21. D	33. A
10. D	22. C	34. D
11. B	23. C	35. C
12. B	24. B	36. B

PART III: SCIENCE

1. D	19. B	37. A
2. A	20. C	38. A
3. C	21. D	39. B
4. D	22. B	40. B
5. D	23. C	41. C
6. C	24. B	42. D
7. A	25. A	43. D
8. B	26. C	44. B
9. A	27. A	45. A
10. D	28. C	46. A
11. B	29. A	47. B
12. A	30. D	48. C
13. B	31. B	49. B
14. A	32. C	50. C
15. D	33. A	51. B
16. A	34. D	52. A
17. B	35. C	53. A
18. C	36. C	

PART IV: ENGLISH AND LANGUAGE USAGE

1. B	11. D	21. C
2. A	12. A	22. A
3. C	13. A	23. C
4. A	14. D	24. C
5. C	15. A	25. D
6. B	16. C	26. A
7. C	17. B	27. B
8. B	18. D	28. C
9. C	19. A	
10. B	20. B	

TEAS Practice Test 2: Explanatory Answers

PART I: READING

1. (C) An encyclopedia (choice A) would be unlikely to include such details as the opening and closing times, but a tourist brochure certainly would.

2. (A) The paragraph tells about the museum's past, present, and future.

3. (A) Both *fascinating* and *user-friendly* are terms designed to interest and win over the reader.

4. (A) The museum is open seven days a week until 5 P.M., so visitors could indeed visit on Sunday afternoon. Documentaries (choice B) are only shown until 3:30; Mardi Gras (choice C) is definitely a holiday, and the museum closes at 5, so it is not open at night (choice D).

5. (B) Because it is meant to inform, the brochure is expository.

6. (B) Just because three particular weeks are mentioned does not mean these are the only days off during the year (choice A). The breaks mentioned are a week apiece, so Spring Break is no longer than the others (choice D). There is no support for choice C.

7. (C) The first, second, and fourth sentences could be proved or checked, but the third is the author's feeling, not a fact.

8. (D) Most of the paragraphs are informative, but the final paragraph includes opinions.

9. (D) This sentence summarizes and adds a personal opinion.

10. (B) According to the passage, such events are included if they "might call for student attendance." The only one that seems to meet that criterion is choice B.

11. (B) The title is quite generic and simply reports on the topic of the passage.

12. (A) Choice A represents the author's essential reason for writing this passage. Readers would read it to learn about those features and functions.

13. (C) The passage is short, but it contains some key plot points. The sultan's motivation is that he wants to add to his treasure. For this reason, he calls upon the wise men. It is logical that he calls upon them for advice.

14. (B) The characters, setting, and plot are typical of certain folktales.

15. (D) An owner's manual contains information on the features of the car.

16. (D) Draw a picture if it helps. After step 1, you are one block east of your starting point. After step 2, you are one block east and two blocks south. After step 3, you are three blocks east and two blocks south.

17. (C) The third test offered in Teeburg is on August 19 and 20. The tests are Friday and Saturday, so August 19 is a Friday. If the application is due the Friday prior to the test, it must be due August 12.

18. (B) To absolve someone is to declare him or her free and clear of blame.

19. (C) A blender is kitchen equipment and would be found at a kitchen equipment store.

20. (B) Canto's ad suggests that they have one-day turnaround on laboratory items.

21. (A) The pulse rate is indicated by the abbreviation *PUL* on the monitor.

22. (C) You should not have to do the math here; it requires only a simple estimate. The two income tax figures add up to a little less than $100. That would be approaching 20 percent.

23. (A) Find the choice that best substitutes for *principally* in the definition in the text: A fat that is solid at room temperature and comes _____ from animal food products and selected plants. The only synonymous substitution is *mostly*.

24. (B) Although *selected* may mean many things, in this context, it simply means "particular" or "certain."

25. (C) The purpose of the passage as a whole is to tout shoes that simulate running barefoot.

26. (B) This is the main idea of the passage—that certain shoes give you the sensation of running barefoot while protecting your feet.

27. (C) A broken water main is news and may require a reporter's coverage.

28. (B) From the airport, the first stop is a local stop, and the second stop is the convention center.

29. (C) There are three local stops between the two express stops at the mall and the museum.

30. (C) Einstein was a far more recent personage than any of the others on this list.

31. (C) First look for the stores that carry turtlenecks: choices B, C, and D. Then look for those that carry blue turtlenecks: choices C and D. Finally find the one that has size M: choice C.

32. (B) Study guides are designed to prepare students for test-taking.

33. (D) Menarche and menopause would be appropriate topics under human reproduction. Since those topics are found on pages 278 through 281, the chapter must encompass those page numbers.

34. (B) Rotating the shape 90 degrees to the right would result in a diagram with triangle 2 pointing left and triangle 1 pointing right. Removing section 1 would leave triangle 2 pointing left. Then step 3 involves drawing a circle around that left-facing triangle.

35. (D) A connotation is an emotional or cultural meaning attached to a word, apart from its dictionary definition. In this case, *uneven* describes a gait that would not be desirable for a marathoner. Therefore, it has a negative connotation in this context.

36. (C) The battle in question must fit the overlying topic of the Civil War. Waterloo (choice A) was a battle of the Napoleonic Wars. Thermopylae (choice B) was a battle of the Greco-Persian Wars. Bunker Hill (choice D) was a battle of the American Revolution. The Siege of Vicksburg (choice C) was a decisive Union victory in the Civil War.

37. (D) *Coverage* has multiple meanings, but only choice D refers to its insurance context.

38. (B) Ms. Jameson says that the new plan is "substantially superior to other plans we have reviewed." She may simply be trying to garner the 30 applicants needed, but her bias seems to be in favor of the plan.

39. (D) The topic (choice A) is "Serpent's Tongue," the main idea (B) is something like "Serpent's Tongue is a useful spring herb," and the theme (choice C) might be "natural remedies." The comparison shown is a detail.

40. (B) Under "Government and virtues," the author describes how the herb works based on the influences of moon and planets on the body.

41. (B) Follow step by step: After step 2, you have 8 ounces of water. After step 3, you have 4 ounces left. After step 4, you have 10 ounces. After step 5, you have 9 ounces.

42. (A) The fastest way to learn this would be to look under *P* for *Patton* in the index of the book.

43. (A) Degrees Celsius are on the left side of this thermometer. The column indicates a temperature of about 24 degrees Celsius.

44. (D) According to the label, a serving gives the consumer 10 percent of the daily requirement of vitamin C, so he has 90 percent yet to consume to equal 100 percent in all.

45. (A) The amount of sodium on the label is 4 percent of a 2,000-calorie diet. In a 1,500-calorie diet, it would represent a greater percent.

46. (A) The darkest bar represents week 1. Plant A has the tallest bar.

47. (B) To answer this, look at the differences in height between week 0 and week 1 bars for each plant, between week 1 and week 2 bars for each plant, and between week 2 and week 3 bars for each plant. In each case, the growth was greatest in week 2.

48. (B) *Mold* has many meanings, but here it means "cast" or "form."

49. (C) The author's argument is that voting ought to be mandatory. The only choice that supports that argument is choice C, which offers another reason that mandatory voting might be a positive move.

50. (B) The conclusion must follow directly from the argument. The author is saying that mandatory voting could have a variety of positive results, including ridding the system of restrictions to voting, thus making it fairer, and including everybody's choice, thus making it more representative.

51. (C) The doctor's dropping of the beaker led to the result or consequence that the room was closed. Other possible words and phrases include *consequently, subsequently,* or *therefore.*

52. (A) A fact can be proved or checked. The other choices all include feelings (*glad, terrifying, distressing*) that cannot be proved.

53. (B) *Casus belli* is Latin for "cause of war." All of the choices name possible reasons to use italics, but only choice B applies here.

Part II: Mathematics

1. (C) Decimals are expressed as tenths, hundredths, and so on. Think: $\frac{2}{5} = \frac{x}{10}$. The answer is 4, so the decimal is 0.4.

2. (B) Add to find the total sold, and divide by 4 hours to find the average per hour: $\frac{24 + 30 + 45 + 17}{4} = \frac{116}{4} = 29$.

3. (A) Find the total amount she spent by multiplying number of stamps by cost: $20 \times \$0.29 = \$5.80$, and $40 \times \$0.42 = \$16.80$. $\$16.80 + \$5.80 = \$22.60$. $\$25.00 - \$22.60 = \$2.40$.

4. (B) Ordinarily, multiplying two numbers with two digits right of the decimal point would result in a product with four digits to the right of the decimal point. Here, however, the last digit, zero, is dropped off.

5. (D) If 1 meter = 3.28 feet, then 6 meters = 3.28 × 6 feet, or 19.68 feet.

6. (D) Think of this as a proportion: $\frac{1 \text{ hour}}{80 \text{ miles}} = \frac{x \text{ hours}}{140 \text{ miles}}$. Cross-multiply to solve: $140 = 80x$; $x = \frac{140}{80}$, or 1.75 hours, which equals 1 hour 45 minutes.

7. (A) Solve by multiplying the cost of the house by 8%: $\$152,000 \times 0.08 = \$12,160$.

8. (B) Multiply the unknowns first: $x \times x = x^2$. Then multiply $3 \times x$ and $x \times 3$, for a total of $3x + 3x$, or $6x$. Finally, multiply 3×3.

9. (B) The formula for circumference of a circle is $2\pi r$. Use 3.14 as an approximation for pi, and the circumference is $2 \times 3 \times 3.14$, or 18.84.

10. (D) The child with the greatest weight gain between birth and 2 months will have the greatest difference between the first and third bars on the graph. A simple visual assessment should prove that child D is that child.

11. (B) Read down and across to find mileage between cities. The distance between Buffalo and Flushing is 370 miles. The distance between Buffalo and Syracuse is 152 miles. $370 - 152 = 218$.

12. (B) First, find the lowest common denominator. $\dfrac{2}{15} \times \dfrac{4}{4} = \dfrac{8}{60}$. $\dfrac{1}{12} \times \dfrac{5}{5} = \dfrac{5}{60}$. $\dfrac{8}{60} + \dfrac{5}{60} = \dfrac{13}{60}$.

13. (D) Despite knowing the range, the only other thing you know for sure is the definition of *median*, which is expressed in choice D.

14. (B) Since each number has one digit after the decimal point, the product should have two digits following the decimal point.

15. (A) 1,000 milliliters = 1 liter, so 2,500 milliliters = 2.5 liters.

16. (C) Look only at the bars for June, July, and August. The sales are $120 + 150 + 100$, for a total of 370.

17. (C) Find out how much one retiree would save: $\$7.00 - \$5.50 = \$1.50$. Now multiply that by 20 to find the total saved: $20 \times \$1.50 = \$30.00$.

18. (D) Express each mixed number as an improper fraction: $\dfrac{21}{4} - \dfrac{23}{6}$. Then find the lowest common denominator and restate those fractions: $\dfrac{126}{24} - \dfrac{92}{24}$. Solve, and express as a mixed number in lowest terms: $\dfrac{34}{24} = 1\dfrac{10}{24} = 1\dfrac{5}{12}$.

19. (A) $12 + 8 = 20$, and $20 - 6 = 14$.

20. (B) The dependent variable is the one whose changes depend on the independent variable. In this case, deepness of voice depends on time.

21. (D) Since you know that $4^2 = 16$, you can rule out choices A and B. Solving the multiplications should show you that $4.2 \times 4.2 = 17.64$, which is close, but not as close as $4.25 \times 4.25 = 18.0625$.

22. (C) Round $895 to $900 and multiply by 20 to find the closest estimate.

23. (C) Express the mixed numbers as improper fractions, and multiply the first by the reciprocal of the second. $4\dfrac{5}{8} = \dfrac{37}{8}$. $1\dfrac{1}{2} = \dfrac{3}{2}$. $\dfrac{37}{8} \times \dfrac{2}{3} = \dfrac{74}{24}$. Now reduce to lowest terms and express the answer as a mixed number. $\dfrac{74}{24} = \dfrac{37}{12} = 3\dfrac{1}{12}$.

24. (B) George paid $3 for the first hour and $1 for each of the three half-hour periods after that. $\$3 + \$1 + \$1 + 1 = \$6$.

25. (C) If James paid $1.44 for 6 lemons, each lemon cost $\$\dfrac{1.44}{6}$, or $0.24. Divide that into $4.80 to find how many Casey bought: $\dfrac{\$4.80}{\$0.24} = 20$.

26. (B) Multiply the xs first to get x^2. Then multiply $5 \times x$ and $1 \times x$ for a total of $6x$. Finally, multiply 5×1.

27. (B) In other words, $75\%x = 18$, or $0.75x = 18$. Solve by dividing both sides by 0.75: $x = \dfrac{18}{0.75}$, or $x = 24$.

28. (C) If 1 inch = 6 inches, 6 inches = 36 inches, or 1 yard.

29. (D) Think about nests you have seen. The twigs are tightly connected. The smallest tool possible would be the best one to use.

30. (D) Read this as "the absolute value of 5 plus the absolute value of negative 3." Absolute value is always a positive number.

31. (D) Call the given number n. Half of that number is $\dfrac{n}{2}$. Four more than that is $\dfrac{n}{2} + 4$.

32. (B) The square root of 9 is 3, 3% is 0.03, and $\dfrac{14}{4}$ is 3.5. Clearly 3% is the least number listed, and $\dfrac{14}{4}$ is the greatest.

33. (A) Change over time is usually best expressed via a line graph.

34. (D) If Olivia is guaranteed 125 hours of lifeguarding time at \$18 per hour, she will make 125 × \$18, or \$2,250, from lifeguarding alone. That leaves \$2,250 more to reach her goal, and \$2,250 ÷ \$15/hour = 150 hours.

35. (C) Look at various ordered pairs on the graph, or simply observe the direction of the data. As the x-values increase, so do the y-values—not by a constant amount, but enough to be considered a positive correlation.

36. (B) Presumably, the prices on the tickets differ, meaning that one price is variable x, and the other is variable y. Since Janelle bought 1 of x and 3 of y, the cost in all would be $x + 3y$.

Part III: Science

1. (D) The esophagus is toward the upper end of the body compared to the stomach, making it superior.

2. (A) Something that is anterior is toward the front of the body. The nose is the most anterior feature on the list of choices.

3. (C) The comparison of results to the original hypothesis takes place as you analyze the data.

4. (D) The arteries carry blood away from the heart as a key feature of the cardiovascular system.

5. (D) The alveoli are the tiny air sacs in the lungs where the exchange of oxygen and carbon dioxide takes place.

6. (C) The ribs themselves protect the lungs (choice A), but the intercostals are muscles that expand and contract the chest, allowing it to draw in and expel air.

7. (A) The root *meter* means "measure." Any of these items, which measure distance, time, and sound, might be used to collect quantitative data.

8. (B) Reading the chart clockwise from top left, the cross is predicted to yield one female carrier, one female hemophiliac, one male hemophiliac, and one normal male.

9. (A) At point X, transcription is "unzipping" DNA to form a strand of mRNA that then creates a protein through translation (choice B).

10. (D) By 5 hours in, the change in population growth has ceased, making $\Delta N = 0$.

11. (B) Only this choice presents you with the control group and test group needed for a valid experiment.

12. (A) Since the point of the experiment is to compare pollution levels at various depths in a lake, only this choice continues the experiment. There is no indication that the experimenter is interested in pollution in saltwater (choice B) or over time (choice D).

13. (B) Peristalsis is the radial contraction and relaxation of muscles that create a wave down a muscular tube; for example, propelling food through the esophagus (as in the diagram) or the small intestine.

14. (A) Sunlight is the primary source of vitamin D in humans—ultraviolet photons are absorbed by 7-dehydrocholesterol in the skin, leading to its transformation to previtamin D_3, which is rapidly converted to vitamin D_3.

15. (D) Scurvy was once the disease of sailors, because months at sea without fruits and vegetables led to vitamin C deficiency. Without vitamin C, the human body cannot synthesize collagen, leading to spongy tissue and bleeding sores.

16. (A) The mass remains the same, at 1 kilogram. Because the volume is now halved, the density (mass/volume) is doubled.

17. (B) A gas with a greater mass effuses less rapidly than a gas with a lesser mass. Therefore, the gas with less mass would be smelled sooner. Since both gases are odorous, and both do effuse eventually, choices C and D are incorrect.

18. (C) The hippocampi, one on either side of the brain under the cerebral cortex, are associated with emotion, the autonomic nervous system, and memory. Shrinkage of the hippocampi is a key sign of Alzheimer's disease.

19. (B) The process begins with blood delivery to the glomerulus, where it is filtered through the glomerular barrier. After that, the filtered part enters the nephron, and the unfiltered part is reabsorbed into the peritubular capillaries.

20. (C) Passive immunity may be achieved through injection, but only injection of antibodies from another person or organism. Vaccines (choices A and B) are examples of active immunity, as is the immunity achieved through exposure to disease (choice D). The natural transfer of antibodies through the placenta, colostrum, or breast milk leads to a temporary form of passive immunity.

21. (D) Reactivity has to do with the tendency of an element to lose electrons. The least reactive elements are the noble gases, and in general, reactivity increases across the periodic table from left to right. Since magnesium and barium are in the same column, they are similar in reactivity.

22. (B) Line II shows a constant death rate, meaning one where age-specific mortality rates are constant.

23. (C) In the example given, year $0 = 1960$. The year 2020, then, is equivalent to year 60 on the graph. At that point on the graph, the species is close to occupying half its potential range. It will fill that range by about the year 2080.

24. (B) During the lag phase, the species has not yet taken hold, and there is still a chance to combat its growth.

25. (A) Fibrin is a protein involved in blood clotting. Connective tissue contains any of three types of protein fibers: collagen, elastic, or reticular. For example, the dense tissue found in tendons is strengthened with collagen fiber, lung tissue contains elastic fiber that gives it flexibility, and adipose tissue is held together by a mesh of reticular fibers.

26. (C) Tap water is relatively neutral and could be expected to fall in that neutral range.

27. (A) A first-degree burn is a superficial burn that affects only the top layer of skin, the epidermis. Second-degree burns may penetrate to the dermis, and third-degree burns may affect deeper tissue.

28. (C) Sebaceous glands in the skin secrete an oily sebum, which lubricates and moisturizes the skin and hair.

29. (A) Splenectomy is the removal of the spleen, usually due to disease or injury. People can live without a spleen, but since the spleen plays a key role in fighting infection, removal of the spleen makes the patient more susceptible to infections of many kinds.

30. (D) The hawk, as a secondary consumer, is at the highest trophic level.

31. (B) If a plant were introduced (choice A), you would expect the number of shrews to increase, because their food supply would increase. If a secondary consumer or predator (choices C and D) were introduced, you might expect the number of snakes to decrease due to competition. However, if a primary consumer similar to the shrew were introduced, competition might kill off the shrew while offering the snake a new source of food.

32. (C) The integumentary system includes the skin, hair, nails, and assorted glands. Receptors embedded in the skin receive information regarding heat, pain, air flow, and so on, which is transported through the nervous system to the brain.

33. (A) Bone tissue stores a variety of minerals, from calcium to phosphorus, releasing them into the bloodstream as needed.

34. (D) Dry ice is frozen carbon dioxide. As it breaks down, it transforms directly into gas without passing through a liquid phase. Sublimation of metals is possible, but not "outside of the laboratory."

35. (C) Because scores do not appear to go up or down when hours of sleep increase or decrease, there is apparently no correlation between the variables.

36. (C) The age (choice A) is not extraneous, as all subjects are kindergarteners. The illness rate (choice B) is not extraneous, and the habitat (choice D), rural and urban, is apparently a point of comparison. There is no differentiation mentioned between boys and girls, implying that gender is an extraneous variable.

37. (A) The upper respiratory tract contains the nasal passages, sinuses, pharynx, and the larynx down to the vocal cords. The laryngopharynx is part of the pharynx.

38. (A) Osteoporosis is a condition in which hormonal changes or mineral deficiencies cause the bones to thin and become brittle. This condition may lead to fractures, curvature of the spine, or compression, any of which may result in height loss. The other diseases mentioned are a skin disease (choice B), a disease of the small intestine (choice C), and an infection of the liver (choice D).

39. (B) The adrenals sit atop the kidneys and produce a variety of hormones, from cortisol and testosterone to epinephrine (adrenaline) and norepinephrine.

40. (B) In the first stage of meiosis, meiosis I, the parent cell splits into two diploid cells. In the second stage, meiosis II, those two cells split to form four haploid cells, each with only one set of chromosomes from the parent cell.

41. (C) Hydrogen bonds between complementary bases (adenine and thymine or cytosine and guanine) stabilize and strengthen the double helix structure of DNA.

42. (D) The seminal vesicles (choice A) and prostate (choice B) produce fluid that combines with sperm cells from the testicles (choice C) to make semen. During ejaculation, that semen is expelled through the urethra.

43. (D) Bears and toads have backbones, so both are in the phylum Chordata (choice B). Starfish are echinoderms, in the phylum Echinodermata. All three are in the kingdom Animalia, however.

44. (B) The lymph nodes are located in the jaw and neck; under the arms and in the chest; in the groin; and in the pelvic cavity, the abdominal cavity, and the thoracic cavity. They are linked by lymphatic vessels and house immune system cells of various kinds. Not only are lymphocytes produced in the nodes, but the nodes also trap and filter out pathogens.

45. (A) As amino acids break down in the process of digestion, that deamination produces ammonia, which could be toxic if left to accumulate. The liver uses enzymes and carrier molecules to convert ammonia and carbon dioxide into urea, which is not quite as harmful and may be removed easily by the kidneys.

46. (A) Smooth muscle tissue lines the blood vessels, stomach, intestines, uterus, and bladder. Most smooth muscle tissue is involuntary, meaning that it is not under conscious control.

47. (B) A suppressor T cell tells the B cell to stop making antibodies, whereas a helper T cell tells it to start.

48. (C) The epiglottis is a flap of cartilage that covers the windpipe during the activity of swallowing.

49. (B) The right atrium receives the "used," or deoxygenated, blood from the body and pumps it to the right ventricle, from which it moves through the pulmonary artery to the lungs. Once it is oxygenated, it returns to the heart via the pulmonary veins through the left atrium, to the left ventricle and out through the aorta to the rest of the body.

50. (C) Amylase begins the process of breaking down starch into sugar.

51. (B) The autonomic (choice B) nervous system is part of the peripheral (choice D) nervous system—the part that is involuntary. It affects such processes as heart rate, digestion, perspiration, and so on. The somatic (choice A) part of the peripheral nervous system is the part that is voluntary.

52. (A) Oxytocin is released from the pituitary to stimulate labor and later initiates the letdown of milk.

53. (A) The crude birth rate is the births per 1,000 organisms per year, and the crude death rate is the deaths per 1,000 organisms per year. If the former far exceeds the latter, overpopulation is possible.

Part IV: English and Language Usage

1. (B) The adverb needed means "at last," and choice B has the correct spelling.

2. (A) The puppy chased the tail belonging to it—its tail. *It's* is a contraction that means *it is*. The correct spelling of *delightedly* is in choice A.

3. (C) The phrase *three days from now* places the action in the future, so the future-tense verb is required.

4. (A) *Iterate* means "to repeat." The correct word is *itinerant*, meaning "traveling from place to place."

5. (C) The predicate is the verb; in this case, *put* (choice C).

6. (B) The pair in choice A are different parts of speech, so they are unlikely to be redundant. Neither pair in choices C and D is really synonymous. Only *adroitness* and *skill* (choice B) name the same quality and can be considered redundant, or repetitive.

7. (C) All of the choices are definitions of *substance*, but only choice C fits the context of the sentence.

8. (B) The conclusion of a paragraph sums up the overall ideas presented in the paragraph. In this case, the order of sentences in the paragraph might logically be A, C, D, B. Choice A is the topic sentence, choices C and D add supporting details, and choice B draws a conclusion about what has come before.

9. (C) In this context, *dish* is a slang word meaning "gossip." *Get together* is idiomatic, but it is not slang.

10. (B) Choices A and D make it seem as though the mother were age seven, and choice C is nonsensical. Only choice B eliminates the problem of misplaced modifiers.

11. (D) The school is not long overdue; the book is.

12. (A) Although choice B is possible if the lunch were made quickly rather than consumed quickly, choice A is far more logical and grammatically correct.

13. (A) The word *staff* may be singular or plural. Here, the pronoun *their* indicates that it is being used as a plural noun, which means that the verb that agrees is *hope* (choice A), not *hopes* (choice B).

14. (D) The action takes place in the future—the time between now and when the semester ends. Therefore, the verb must be in the future tense.

15. (A) The foxes are not ingenuous, meaning "naive." They are ingenious, meaning "clever."

16. (C) The antecedent is the plural noun *animals*, so the pronoun must be third person; because it follows the verb, it must be an object pronoun, *them*.

17. (B) "The following statement" is a clue that this part of the sentence introduces something, making the colon the best choice here.

18. (D) *Too* means "overly," *to* means "on the way toward," and *two* is a number.

19. (A) If you stop to recognize the word's connection to *critic*, you will choose correctly.

20. (B) The suffix *-ize* frequently changes nouns to verbs, as it does in choice B, changing the noun *hospital* to a verb meaning "to place in a hospital." None of the other choices are verbs; choices A and D are nouns, and choice C is an adjective.

21. (C) Mona is asking a question and holding up a flower. The question mark must come within the quotation marks, and the participial phrase should be set off with a comma.

22. (A) To make this passive sentence active, you must insert a new subject to perform the action, in this case, *someone*.

23. (C) *One* (choice A) and *someone* (choice D) are singular and require a singular verb. *Several* (choice B) is plural and requires a plural verb. *Either* (choice C) is always singular and takes a singular verb.

24. (C) Only choice C is a word.

25. (D) Although *mangled* may be a verb (choice B), it is used here to modify *wing* and is thus an adjective (choice C).

26. (A) Choices B and D capitalize unimportant words. Choice C fails to capitalize important words. Only choice A follows the rules for capitalization of book titles.

27. (B) A simple sentence may have a compound subject or a compound predicate, but it will never have two separate subject and predicate combinations. Sentences A, C, and D are complex; each contains a dependent clause as well as the primary independent clause.

28. (C) *Ante-* means "before"; we use it to speak of the period before the Civil War, which we call *antebellum*. *Natal*, with the same root as *nativity*, means "birth."

TEAS PRACTICE TEST 3

TEAS Practice Test 3: Answer Sheet

READING

1 (A) (B) (C) (D)	19 (A) (B) (C) (D)	37 (A) (B) (C) (D)
2 (A) (B) (C) (D)	20 (A) (B) (C) (D)	38 (A) (B) (C) (D)
3 (A) (B) (C) (D)	21 (A) (B) (C) (D)	39 (A) (B) (C) (D)
4 (A) (B) (C) (D)	22 (A) (B) (C) (D)	40 (A) (B) (C) (D)
5 (A) (B) (C) (D)	23 (A) (B) (C) (D)	41 (A) (B) (C) (D)
6 (A) (B) (C) (D)	24 (A) (B) (C) (D)	42 (A) (B) (C) (D)
7 (A) (B) (C) (D)	25 (A) (B) (C) (D)	43 (A) (B) (C) (D)
8 (A) (B) (C) (D)	26 (A) (B) (C) (D)	44 (A) (B) (C) (D)
9 (A) (B) (C) (D)	27 (A) (B) (C) (D)	45 (A) (B) (C) (D)
10 (A) (B) (C) (D)	28 (A) (B) (C) (D)	46 (A) (B) (C) (D)
11 (A) (B) (C) (D)	29 (A) (B) (C) (D)	47 (A) (B) (C) (D)
12 (A) (B) (C) (D)	30 (A) (B) (C) (D)	48 (A) (B) (C) (D)
13 (A) (B) (C) (D)	31 (A) (B) (C) (D)	49 (A) (B) (C) (D)
14 (A) (B) (C) (D)	32 (A) (B) (C) (D)	50 (A) (B) (C) (D)
15 (A) (B) (C) (D)	33 (A) (B) (C) (D)	51 (A) (B) (C) (D)
16 (A) (B) (C) (D)	34 (A) (B) (C) (D)	52 (A) (B) (C) (D)
17 (A) (B) (C) (D)	35 (A) (B) (C) (D)	53 (A) (B) (C) (D)
18 (A) (B) (C) (D)	36 (A) (B) (C) (D)	

MATHEMATICS

1 (A) (B) (C) (D)	13 (A) (B) (C) (D)	25 (A) (B) (C) (D)
2 (A) (B) (C) (D)	14 (A) (B) (C) (D)	26 (A) (B) (C) (D)
3 (A) (B) (C) (D)	15 (A) (B) (C) (D)	27 (A) (B) (C) (D)
4 (A) (B) (C) (D)	16 (A) (B) (C) (D)	28 (A) (B) (C) (D)
5 (A) (B) (C) (D)	17 (A) (B) (C) (D)	29 (A) (B) (C) (D)
6 (A) (B) (C) (D)	18 (A) (B) (C) (D)	30 (A) (B) (C) (D)
7 (A) (B) (C) (D)	19 (A) (B) (C) (D)	31 (A) (B) (C) (D)
8 (A) (B) (C) (D)	20 (A) (B) (C) (D)	32 (A) (B) (C) (D)
9 (A) (B) (C) (D)	21 (A) (B) (C) (D)	33 (A) (B) (C) (D)
10 (A) (B) (C) (D)	22 (A) (B) (C) (D)	34 (A) (B) (C) (D)
11 (A) (B) (C) (D)	23 (A) (B) (C) (D)	35 (A) (B) (C) (D)
12 (A) (B) (C) (D)	24 (A) (B) (C) (D)	36 (A) (B) (C) (D)

SCIENCE

1	Ⓐ	Ⓑ	Ⓒ	Ⓓ	19	Ⓐ	Ⓑ	Ⓒ	Ⓓ	37	Ⓐ	Ⓑ	Ⓒ	Ⓓ
2	Ⓐ	Ⓑ	Ⓒ	Ⓓ	20	Ⓐ	Ⓑ	Ⓒ	Ⓓ	38	Ⓐ	Ⓑ	Ⓒ	Ⓓ
3	Ⓐ	Ⓑ	Ⓒ	Ⓓ	21	Ⓐ	Ⓑ	Ⓒ	Ⓓ	39	Ⓐ	Ⓑ	Ⓒ	Ⓓ
4	Ⓐ	Ⓑ	Ⓒ	Ⓓ	22	Ⓐ	Ⓑ	Ⓒ	Ⓓ	40	Ⓐ	Ⓑ	Ⓒ	Ⓓ
5	Ⓐ	Ⓑ	Ⓒ	Ⓓ	23	Ⓐ	Ⓑ	Ⓒ	Ⓓ	41	Ⓐ	Ⓑ	Ⓒ	Ⓓ
6	Ⓐ	Ⓑ	Ⓒ	Ⓓ	24	Ⓐ	Ⓑ	Ⓒ	Ⓓ	42	Ⓐ	Ⓑ	Ⓒ	Ⓓ
7	Ⓐ	Ⓑ	Ⓒ	Ⓓ	25	Ⓐ	Ⓑ	Ⓒ	Ⓓ	43	Ⓐ	Ⓑ	Ⓒ	Ⓓ
8	Ⓐ	Ⓑ	Ⓒ	Ⓓ	26	Ⓐ	Ⓑ	Ⓒ	Ⓓ	44	Ⓐ	Ⓑ	Ⓒ	Ⓓ
9	Ⓐ	Ⓑ	Ⓒ	Ⓓ	27	Ⓐ	Ⓑ	Ⓒ	Ⓓ	45	Ⓐ	Ⓑ	Ⓒ	Ⓓ
10	Ⓐ	Ⓑ	Ⓒ	Ⓓ	28	Ⓐ	Ⓑ	Ⓒ	Ⓓ	46	Ⓐ	Ⓑ	Ⓒ	Ⓓ
11	Ⓐ	Ⓑ	Ⓒ	Ⓓ	29	Ⓐ	Ⓑ	Ⓒ	Ⓓ	47	Ⓐ	Ⓑ	Ⓒ	Ⓓ
12	Ⓐ	Ⓑ	Ⓒ	Ⓓ	30	Ⓐ	Ⓑ	Ⓒ	Ⓓ	48	Ⓐ	Ⓑ	Ⓒ	Ⓓ
13	Ⓐ	Ⓑ	Ⓒ	Ⓓ	31	Ⓐ	Ⓑ	Ⓒ	Ⓓ	49	Ⓐ	Ⓑ	Ⓒ	Ⓓ
14	Ⓐ	Ⓑ	Ⓒ	Ⓓ	32	Ⓐ	Ⓑ	Ⓒ	Ⓓ	50	Ⓐ	Ⓑ	Ⓒ	Ⓓ
15	Ⓐ	Ⓑ	Ⓒ	Ⓓ	33	Ⓐ	Ⓑ	Ⓒ	Ⓓ	51	Ⓐ	Ⓑ	Ⓒ	Ⓓ
16	Ⓐ	Ⓑ	Ⓒ	Ⓓ	34	Ⓐ	Ⓑ	Ⓒ	Ⓓ	52	Ⓐ	Ⓑ	Ⓒ	Ⓓ
17	Ⓐ	Ⓑ	Ⓒ	Ⓓ	35	Ⓐ	Ⓑ	Ⓒ	Ⓓ	53	Ⓐ	Ⓑ	Ⓒ	Ⓓ
18	Ⓐ	Ⓑ	Ⓒ	Ⓓ	36	Ⓐ	Ⓑ	Ⓒ	Ⓓ					

ENGLISH AND LANGUAGE USAGE

1	Ⓐ	Ⓑ	Ⓒ	Ⓓ	11	Ⓐ	Ⓑ	Ⓒ	Ⓓ	21	Ⓐ	Ⓑ	Ⓒ	Ⓓ
2	Ⓐ	Ⓑ	Ⓒ	Ⓓ	12	Ⓐ	Ⓑ	Ⓒ	Ⓓ	22	Ⓐ	Ⓑ	Ⓒ	Ⓓ
3	Ⓐ	Ⓑ	Ⓒ	Ⓓ	13	Ⓐ	Ⓑ	Ⓒ	Ⓓ	23	Ⓐ	Ⓑ	Ⓒ	Ⓓ
4	Ⓐ	Ⓑ	Ⓒ	Ⓓ	14	Ⓐ	Ⓑ	Ⓒ	Ⓓ	24	Ⓐ	Ⓑ	Ⓒ	Ⓓ
5	Ⓐ	Ⓑ	Ⓒ	Ⓓ	15	Ⓐ	Ⓑ	Ⓒ	Ⓓ	25	Ⓐ	Ⓑ	Ⓒ	Ⓓ
6	Ⓐ	Ⓑ	Ⓒ	Ⓓ	16	Ⓐ	Ⓑ	Ⓒ	Ⓓ	26	Ⓐ	Ⓑ	Ⓒ	Ⓓ
7	Ⓐ	Ⓑ	Ⓒ	Ⓓ	17	Ⓐ	Ⓑ	Ⓒ	Ⓓ	27	Ⓐ	Ⓑ	Ⓒ	Ⓓ
8	Ⓐ	Ⓑ	Ⓒ	Ⓓ	18	Ⓐ	Ⓑ	Ⓒ	Ⓓ	28	Ⓐ	Ⓑ	Ⓒ	Ⓓ
9	Ⓐ	Ⓑ	Ⓒ	Ⓓ	19	Ⓐ	Ⓑ	Ⓒ	Ⓓ					
10	Ⓐ	Ⓑ	Ⓒ	Ⓓ	20	Ⓐ	Ⓑ	Ⓒ	Ⓓ					

Part I. Reading

53 questions (47 scored), 64 minutes

Semi-Formal

Watching her younger sister prepare for the semi-formal dance gave Teresa an unfamiliar feeling. Claudia was so mature compared to Teresa at that age, she thought. Teresa had been shy and studious, with her nose in a book at all times. Claudia's grades were fine, but her social life was exceptional.

"Help me pick out a dress," Claudia urged her sister. For Claudia to show any sort of insecurity was rare. Teresa felt warm inside to think that her sister might be relying on her taste.

"Sure," she responded. "I'll drive you up to the mall tomorrow."

At the mall, Claudia disappeared into the dressing room with an armful of possibilities. Teresa went from rack to rack, touching the spangled materials. From time to time, Claudia would come out and twirl, but nothing seemed to be the perfect dress of her semi-formal fantasies.

At the back of the store, Teresa found a silver-gray dress whose fabric was as soft as duck down. Unable to tear herself away, she pulled out the dress and pressed it up against her winter coat, turning this way and that and imagining what it might be like to wear such a beautiful thing.

"Ooh, I love it! It's so different!" cried Claudia, snatching the dress from Teresa's hands. "I knew you would find me the perfect dress. You have such a good eye!"

Teresa smiled at the compliment, watching wistfully as Claudia paraded out wearing the silver confection. Obediently, she held Claudia's bags as her sister paid for the beautiful silver dress. Claudia flung her free arm around her sister's shoulders. "Thanks for your help, sis," she said. "I'll buy you lunch."

The next seven questions are based on this passage.

1. Is the following a topic, main idea, supporting detail, or theme of the passage?

   Jealousy

   A) Topic
   B) Main idea
   C) Supporting detail
   D) Theme

GO ON TO THE NEXT PAGE

---

2. Which of the following is the author's intention in writing this passage?

A) To inform
B) To persuade
C) To entertain
D) To reflect

3. What is a logical conclusion to draw from the fifth paragraph?

A) Teresa thinks the dress is perfect for her sister.
B) Teresa wants the gray dress for herself.
C) Teresa picked a dress her sister will not like.
D) Teresa expects to go to the dance in that dress.

4. Which of the following excerpts from the passage contains an opinion?

A) At the mall, Claudia disappeared into the dressing room with an armful of possibilities.
B) Claudia was so mature compared to Teresa at that age, she thought.
C) Teresa went from rack to rack, touching the spangled materials.
D) Claudia flung her free arm around her sister's shoulders.

5. Which of the following inferences may logically be drawn from the passage?

A) The sisters get along but are not very similar.
B) The sisters are fairly similar but do not get along.
C) The sisters get along because they are so similar.
D) The sisters are quite different and do not get along.

6. The passage is reflective of which of the following types of writing?

A) Narrative
B) Expository
C) Technical
D) Persuasive

7. Which of the following sentences represents a topic sentence for the passage?

A) Watching her younger sister prepare for the semi-formal dance gave Teresa an unfamiliar feeling.
B) From time to time, Claudia would come out and twirl, but nothing seemed to be the perfect dress of her semi-formal fantasies.
C) Teresa smiled at the compliment, watching wistfully as Claudia paraded out wearing the silver confection.
D) At the back of the store, Teresa found a silver-gray dress whose fabric was as soft as duck down.

GO ON TO THE NEXT PAGE

The Pro Side of Termites

We tend to view termites only in terms of their destructive potential, but perhaps it is time to think of their potential for good. Yes, they are agricultural pests and cause millions of dollars in damage to wood structures, but perhaps they have some useful properties as well.

It may come as a shock to you to learn that in certain cultures, termites are part of the human diet. In parts of Africa and southern Asia, people eat winged termites roasted or fried (after first removing their wings). They are said to have a nutty taste and to be rich in protein.

Termites are important in other ways. They create habitats for other species, whether by hollowing trees or by building large termite mounds. They clear away flammable materials on the savanna, lessening the possibility of grass fire. In addition, termites are notoriously efficient energy-producers. They break down wood products quickly, releasing hydrogen as they do so. Scientists are studying their biochemical processes in hopes of reproducing them on a large scale as a source of renewable energy.

The next five questions are based on this passage.

8. Which of the following is the author's main purpose for writing this passage?

   A) To compare the destructive habits of termites with those of other species
   B) To persuade citizens to stop the wanton eradication of termites
   C) To appeal to human forgiveness through a poignant story about termites
   D) To suggest that a destructive creature may have constructive qualities as well

9. Which of the following conclusions may be drawn directly from the second paragraph of the passage?

   A) The author has actually tasted roasted or fried termites.
   B) The author has heard about the consumption of termites.
   C) The author does not believe that people ever eat termites.
   D) The author is disgusted by the notion of eating termites.

10. The passage is reflective of which of the following types of writing?

   A) Technical
   B) Narrative
   C) Descriptive
   D) Expository

GO ON TO THE NEXT PAGE

11. Which of the following statements best describes the author's bias?

A) She is biased against termites.
B) She thinks termites are both good and bad.
C) She approves of everything termites do.
D) She is biased in favor of termites.

12. The author's list of termites' uses in the final paragraph is reflective of which of the following types of text structure?

A) Opinion and examples
B) Problem-solution
C) Comparison-contrast
D) Space order

Recall policy: FDA has no authority to order a recall of a cosmetic, although it can request that a firm recall a product. However, we do have an active role in recalls. For example:

- We monitor the progress of a recall. In addition to reviewing firm status reports, we may conduct our own <u>audit checks</u> at wholesale or retail customers to verify the recall's effectiveness.
- We evaluate the health hazard presented by the product under recall and assign a classification to indicate the degree of hazard posed by a product under recall.

The next two questions are based on this passage.

13. What is an audit check?

A) A restraint on appraisals
B) Payment for inventory
C) A test of hearing
D) A review or inspection

14. A recall policy is a policy involving

A) the ability to remember.
B) the withdrawal of products.
C) the manufacture of cosmetics.
D) the effectiveness of customers.

GO ON TO THE NEXT PAGE

Eleanor Roosevelt was more than just a First Lady. Following her husband's death, she became a world-renowned author, speaker, and political activist. Although her name was presented as a possible running mate for Harry Truman, she chose not to run for public office. She spoke in favor of the United Nations and was a delegate there for five years. Later, she chaired the Presidential Commission on the Status of Women.

The next two questions are based on this passage.

15. Eleanor Roosevelt was more than just a First Lady.

   In the context of the paragraph, does this sentence constitute a topic, a main idea, a theme, or supporting details?

   A) Topic
   B) Main idea
   C) Theme
   D) Supporting details

16. What is the author's apparent purpose for writing this paragraph about Eleanor Roosevelt?

   A) To explain her background
   B) To list her accomplishments
   C) To express personal feelings
   D) To entertain the reader

GO ON TO THE NEXT PAGE

Nutrition Facts

Serving size 1 tsp. (6 g)
Servings about 60

Amount/serving	
Calories 15	Calories from fat 0

	% Daily value*
Total fat 0 g	0%
Saturated fat 0 g	0%
Trans fat 0 g	
Cholesterol 0 mg	0%
Sodium 60 mg	3%
Total carbohydrate 3 g	1%
Dietary fiber 0 g	0%
Sugars 3 g	
Protein 0 g	

Vitamin A 0%	•	Vitamin C 0%	
Calcium 0%	•	Iron 0%	

• Percent daily values are based on a 2,000 calorie diet.

REFRIGERATE AFTER OPENING
INGREDIENTS: Yellow mustard (vinegar, water, no. 1 grade mustard seed, salt, turmeric), sugar, cider, vinegar, aged cayenne pepper, naturally brewed soy sauce (water, soybeans, wheat, salt), tomato paste, molasses, spices, natural smoke flavor.
CONTAINS ALLERGENS: Soy, wheat.

The next two questions are based on this chart.

17. Why should someone with a gluten allergy stay away from this product?

   A) It contains wheat.
   B) It contains sodium.
   C) It contains no fat.
   D) It contains sugar.

18. Based on the ingredients, where would you expect to find this product?

   A) In the dairy case
   B) With sauces and ketchups
   C) In the produce department
   D) With baked goods

GO ON TO THE NEXT PAGE

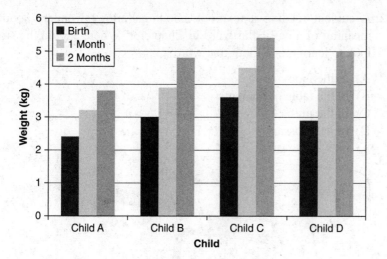

The next two questions are based on this graph.

19. What was the birth weight of the smallest newborn?

    A) 2.1 kg
    B) 2.4 kg
    C) 2.9 kg
    D) 3.4 kg

20. At the end of two months, the difference in weight between the heaviest and lightest child was about

    A) 1 kg.
    B) 1.5 kg.
    C) 2 kg.
    D) 2.5 kg.

21. Read and follow the directions below.

    1. Imagine a canvas divided into 12 vertical sections.
    2. Beginning with the first section, paint every other section blue.
    3. Beginning with the second section, paint every other section white.
    4. Paint every third section red.

    How many sections will be painted only white?

    A) 2 sections
    B) 4 sections
    C) 6 sections
    D) 8 sections

GO ON TO THE NEXT PAGE

22. A student reading a textbook about pathology wonders about the meaning of a particular word in Chapter 1. Where should the student look to learn more about that word?

A) In the index
B) In the table of contents
C) In the preface
D) In the glossary

23.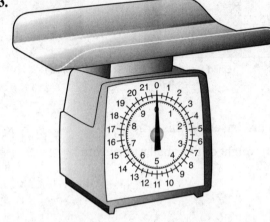

On this scale, a weight of 9 pounds is about equal to a weight of

A) 4 grams.
B) 20 grams.
C) 4 kilograms.
D) 20 kilograms.

The following e-mail was sent by a head nurse to the nurses under her supervision.

Everyone—

Please note that new regulations for sanitation require us to use the hallway sanitizers *every time* we enter a patient's room and again after leaving the room. Although this seems like overkill to some folks, there is no such thing as too much protection when it comes to staph and other deadly infectious agents. Failure to follow these regs will result in a note in your file. Thanks.

The next two questions are based on this passage.

24. How does the author feel about the new regulations?

A) They are overly strict.
B) They are not strict enough.
C) They are strict but important.
D) They are not worth following.

GO ON TO THE NEXT PAGE

25. In the context of the e-mail, what does *overkill* mean?

A) Slaughter
B) Spotlessness
C) Heavy-handedness
D) Crushing defeat

26. Lymph
   composition of, 140
   formation of, 139
Lymph nodes, 140
Lymphatic system, 138–140
Lymphocytes, 137, 147

A student wants to learn more about how lymph is formed in the body. Based on this excerpt from a physiology textbook's index, on which of the following pages should the student begin to look?

A) 137
B) 138
C) 139
D) 140

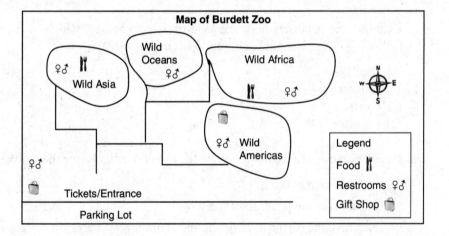

The next two questions are based on this map.

27. A family wants to spend an hour in each section of the zoo. If they start at 9:30 A.M. and hope to eat lunch at a zoo café around noon, in which order should they visit the sections?

A) Wild Asia, Wild Oceans, Wild Africa, Wild Americas
B) Wild Americas, Wild Africa, Wild Oceans, Wild Asia
C) Wild Asia, Wild Africa, Wild Oceans, Wild Americas
D) Wild Oceans, Wild Asia, Wild Americas, Wild Africa

GO ON TO THE NEXT PAGE

28. A tour group starts at the entrance and winds clockwise around the zoo. What is the last section they visit before leaving?

A) A section with a restaurant
B) A section with a gift shop
C) A section with aquatic animals
D) The section farthest from the parking lot

29. Which of these sentences indicates the end of a sequence of events?

A) Moving offstage, James gripped his new diploma and grinned.
B) He shook hands with the dean and took the folder she gave him.
C) James marched into the auditorium with the rest of his class.
D) A few short speeches preceded the calling of graduates' names.

30. Chapter 3: Skin Diseases

   1. Types of Lesions

      A. Nodules
      B. Pustules
      C. Plaques
      D. _____
      E. Ulcers

Examine the headings above. Based on what you see, which of the following is a reasonable heading to insert in the blank spot?

A) Papillae
B) Epidermis
C) Cysts
D) Glands

31. Begin with the word *demon.* Follow the directions to change the word.

   1. Change the *d* to *w*.
   2. Reverse the position of the vowels.
   3. Move the final two letters to the beginning of the word.
   4. Change the *w* to *t*.
   5. Add a *b* to the end of the word.

Which of the following is the new word?

A) women
B) entomb
C) ended
D) womb

GO ON TO THE NEXT PAGE

32. A supporter of a local candidate wants to send a letter to the newspaper telling voters to elect that candidate. Which department of the newspaper should she contact?

    A) Editorial
    B) Business
    C) Local news
    D) Classified

33. Chapter 2: Animal Herbivores

    A. The Seed Eaters
    B. The Predators
    C. The Leaf Nibblers
    D. The Nectar Drinkers

    Analyze the headings above. Which of the following headings is out of place?

    A) The Seed Eaters
    B) The Predators
    C) The Leaf Nibblers
    D) The Nectar Drinkers

34. Which of the following would *not* be considered a primary source?

    A) A speech by an abolitionist
    B) A biography of Harriet Tubman
    C) Clothing from the 1860s
    D) The diary of a freed slave

35. A traveler wants to determine the best place to stay while on the island of Tortola in the British Virgin Islands. Which is the best resource for him to use?

    A) A recent travel guide to the British Virgin Islands
    B) A true crime book called *Trouble in Tortola*
    C) *History of the Virgin Islands*
    D) *The Sugar Mill Caribbean Cookbook*

36. Bill tends to eschew anyone who doesn't conform to his ideals.

    Which of the following is the definition of the word *eschew*?

    A) Steer clear of
    B) Play the part of
    C) Donate to
    D) Be a factor in

GO ON TO THE NEXT PAGE

37. Until we better understand its connotation, let us concentrate on the *denotation* of the word as used in the text.

Why is the word *denotation* italicized in the sentence above?

A) To emphasize the word
B) To indicate use of a foreign term
C) To set off a title
D) To indicate a stage direction

38. For years, mercury was used in thermometers because it is a bright silvery metal that is liquid at room temperature and has a high coefficient of expansion. However, mercury has the disadvantage of being extremely toxic. Although the amount in an oral thermometer is minuscule, the chance of ingesting or inhaling it is enough that the EPA recommends using alternatives in the home. The alcohol thermometer, first used by Daniel Fahrenheit in 1709, is a common household device. Alcohol works in much the same way as mercury, but it has the advantage of being harmless and quickly evaporating if the glass tube is broken. The transparent alcohol is made visible through the addition of red or blue dye.

What do alcohol and mercury have in common?

A) Both are metals.
B) Both may be dyed.
C) Both expand and contract.
D) Neither should be inhaled.

39.

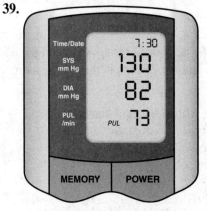

Based on the blood pressure monitor above, which of the following is the patient's pulse rate?

A) 73
B) 82
C) 130
D) $\dfrac{130}{82}$

GO ON TO THE NEXT PAGE

Online Store	Price	Sales Tax	Shipping
Moxie's	$25.95	no	$5.95
Club Y	$24.98	no	$2.98
Joyful	$22.95	yes	$4.25
Shorebird	$24.75	yes	free over $25

40. The chart above gives four possible prices for the same item. If sales tax ranges from 4 to 8 percent, which store offers the best deal?

A) Moxie's
B) Club Y
C) Joyful
D) Shorebird

SMOKE DETECTORS 281

SIGN LANGUAGE

See Translators & Interpreters

Di MARCO SIGNS
Specialists in illumination
and backlighting!
185 Elm St.

SIGNS

American Sign 15 Morton St 555-1284

Carbon Copies 87 Main St 555-2499

Di Marco Signs 185 Elm St 555-3434

Marshall Signs 24 Main St 555-3100

SIGNS—ERECTING & HANGING

American Sign 15 Morton St 555-1284

SIGNS—MAINTENANCE & REPAIR

Di Marco Signs 185 Elm St 555-3434

Marshall Signs 24 Main St 555-3100

SKATING RINKS & PARKS

Cass Park Rink 701 Judd Rd. 555-9411

JM Sports Complex College Pl. . . . .

www.jmcomplex.net 555-1414

SKI INSTRUCTION
Bergen Skis Truxton Blvd . . . 555-3116
Donahue Trails 13 Pine Rd . . . 555-9495
SKIN CARE
Altima Spa 425 Morton St . . . 555-6880
Krystal's on Main 23 Main St . . . 555-8300
SMOKE DETECTORS
Alarm Service 280 Elm St . . . 555-2413

KRYSTAL's ON MAIN STREET
Full-service salon
nails, hair, makeup,
spa services
555-8300, Mon-Sat

The next two questions are based on this sample yellow page.

41. A play producer hopes to find an American Sign Language interpreter to assist with his latest production. What step should he take?

A) Call 555-1284.
B) Turn to *Translators* in the Yellow Pages.
C) Call Information and ask for "Sign Language."
D) Call Krystal's on Main Street.

GO ON TO THE NEXT PAGE

42. On which day is Krystal's on Main Street closed?

A) Monday
B) Thursday
C) Saturday
D) Sunday

43.

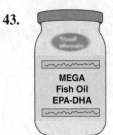

60 geltabs
$15.99/bottle
second bottle 1/2 price

Provides 840 mg of
EPA/DHA per serving
to support the health
of heart, brain, joints,
skin, and more.

If you purchased two bottles of these fish oil pills, you would obtain

A) 120 geltabs for around $24.
B) 60 geltabs for around $24.
C) 120 geltabs for around $32.
D) 60 geltabs for around $32.

44. I appreciate her <u>acumen</u>; her good advice has never steered me wrong.

Which of the following is the definition of the word *acumen*?

A) Zest
B) Interest
C) Insight
D) Gravity

GO ON TO THE NEXT PAGE

"I have called you together," said Inspector Thomas to the family members in the drawing room, "so that I may reveal to you what I have learned. In the course of our discussion, you will discover the identity of the thief as well as the motive behind the theft."

The next two questions are based on this passage.

45. Based on the passage, which of the following is a logical prediction of what the inspector will do?

   A) Ask the family members to close their eyes.
   B) Present his interpretation of a crime.
   C) Allow one or more family members to leave.
   D) Amuse the family with an invented story.

46. Based on a prior knowledge of literature, the reader can infer that this passage was taken from which of the following?

   A) A newspaper article
   B) A narrative poem
   C) A persuasive essay
   D) A detective novel

47. A student skimming *A Field Guide to the Birds* wonders whether it contains information on semipalmated plovers. Where should the student look to learn the answer?

   A) In the index
   B) In the table of contents
   C) In the preface
   D) In the glossary

48. Read and follow the directions below.

   1. Imagine a drawer holding five pairs of socks in five colors—brown, black, green, blue, and red.
   2. Remove one green sock.
   3. Remove one red sock.
   4. Remove two black socks.
   5. Add three green socks.

   Which of the following tells the number of complete pairs of socks now in the drawer?

   A) 3 pairs
   B) 4 pairs
   C) 5 pairs
   D) 6 pairs

GO ON TO THE NEXT PAGE

Glenda Jones <gwh@ps.edu>

Projections   8:45 A.M.

To: Commissioner

Attached please find projections on school enrollment for the local charter (Abbey) and public school in the Hinckley neighborhood. With enrollment capped at 350, there is little fear of overcrowding in the near future. The Abbey numbers could be due to test scores but may also connect to changes along the waterfront, leading to increased traffic and fewer housing units.

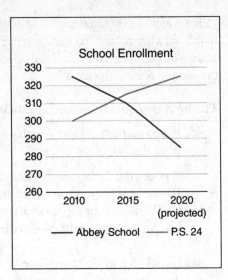

The next two questions are based on this e-mail and graph.

49. What was the population of the charter school in 2010?

    A) 285
    B) 300
    C) 310
    D) 325

50. To draw a conclusion about the reasons for population decline, what might the commissioner want to know about housing unit reductions along the waterfront?

    A) Will any new waterfront housing be built for families?
    B) Did children in those units all attend Abbey School?
    C) Is the increased traffic a result of reduced housing?
    D) How many blocks is P.S. 24 from the waterfront?

GO ON TO THE NEXT PAGE

Visiting the Newseum

The popular Newseum in Washington, DC, was founded in 2008 to illustrate the role of the media in freedom of expression. It is worth a visit both for its stunning exhibits and for its fascinating interactive displays.

Before you enter the museum, be sure to look at the front pages that ring the building. Most people then view the museum from the top down, taking glass elevators to the top, where there is a fabulous view of the city. The Front Pages Gallery continues on the top floor, and you can find newspapers from the early days of publishing all the way up through the present day in the News History Gallery. A video wall shows revolving news broadcasts from important days in history.

A New Media Gallery downstairs lets you test out the latest digital media. Next door, the First Amendment Gallery is a thoughtful reminder of our constitutional rights. The 9/11 Gallery has photographs and artifacts from that terrible day in history.

The other levels of the museum explore freedom of the press around the world, feature an interactive newsroom and 4-D movies, and display Pulitzer-prize-winning news photos from 1917 on. Plan to spend several hours in this enthralling museum.

The next three questions are based on this passage.

51. According to the author, what might you find in the News History Gallery?

    A) An interactive newsroom
    B) A newspaper from the 18th century
    C) Artifacts from important days in history
    D) A display of prize-winning news photographs

52. Based on the article, what should you do just after entering the museum?

    A) Look at the front pages that ring the entrance.
    B) Watch one of the many 4-D movies.
    C) Take an elevator up to see the view.
    D) Test out the latest digital media.

53. Which reason does the author give for recommending the museum?

    A) It explores freedom of the press.
    B) It is popular with visitors of all ages.
    C) It has great interactive displays.
    D) It reminds us of our rights and history.

STOP. THIS IS THE END OF PART I.

Part II. Mathematics

36 items (32 scored), 54 minutes

1. $4\frac{2}{3} \times 6\frac{1}{2}$

   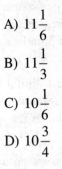

   Simplify the expression above. Which of the following is correct?

   A) $11\frac{1}{6}$

   B) $11\frac{1}{3}$

   C) $10\frac{1}{6}$

   D) $10\frac{3}{4}$

2.

Treatment for	Brand-Name Drug	Generic Drug
High cholesterol	$95/month	$37/month
Arthritis	$135/month	$30/month
Heartburn	$179/month	$15/month

This pharmacy chart shows the costs per month of certain generic versus brand-name medicines.

Over the course of a year, how much could you save by using a generic arthritis medication rather than its brand-name equivalent?

A) $105
B) $360
C) $630
D) $1,260

GO ON TO THE NEXT PAGE

3.

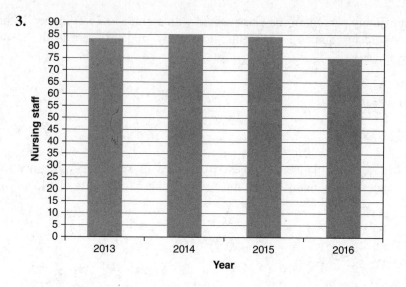

The graph above shows the number of nursing staff at Bedloe Hospital during four years.

Between 2014 and 2016, how many nursing positions were lost?

A) 2
B) 8
C) 10
D) 20

4. Find the total area of the figure shown.

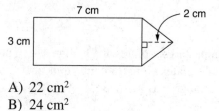

A) 22 cm^2
B) 24 cm^2
C) 27 cm^2
D) 30 cm^2

5. $(4x + 1)(4x - 1)$

Simplify the expression above. Which of the following is correct?

A) $16x^2 - 1$
B) $16x^2 - x - 1$
C) $x - 1$
D) $8x^2 - 1$

GO ON TO THE NEXT PAGE

6. Eighty percent of the class passed with a grade of 75 or higher. If that percent equaled 24 students, how many students were in the whole class?

A) 18
B) 30
C) 36
D) 60

7. If a party planner assumes two bottles of sparkling water per five guests, how many bottles must she purchase for a party of 145?

A) 27
B) 36
C) 49
D) 58

8. How many kilometers are there in 12 miles? (Note: 1 mile = 1.6 kilometers.)

A) 7.5 kilometers
B) 13.2 kilometers
C) 19.2 kilometers
D) 22 kilometers

9. Which answer is correct for the product 0.6×0.55?

A) 0.0033
B) 0.033
C) 0.33
D) 3.3

10. Stu purchased a set of six cups and six plates at a garage sale. The cups were 25 cents apiece, and the plates were 75 cents apiece. If Stu paid with a $10 bill, how much change was he owed?

A) $4.00
B) $4.50
C) $5.00
D) $5.50

11. Stan's scores on five math tests were 87, 92, 87, 88, and 91. What was the mode of this set of data?

A) 87
B) 88
C) 89
D) 90

GO ON TO THE NEXT PAGE

12. Express 1.25 as a fraction in lowest terms.

A) $1\dfrac{1}{25}$

B) $1\dfrac{2}{5}$

C) $1\dfrac{1}{2}$

D) $1\dfrac{1}{4}$

13. $3\dfrac{1}{2} \div 1\dfrac{1}{10}$

Simplify the expression above. Which of the following is correct?

A) $3\dfrac{1}{20}$

B) $3\dfrac{2}{11}$

C) $3\dfrac{1}{5}$

D) $3\dfrac{2}{23}$

14.

Deposits	Withdrawals	Beginning Balance
		$689.98
$1,027.29		
	$40.00	
	$40.00	
	$770.00	
	$40.00	
	$84.75	

This table shows Kyra's checking account during the month of May.

What was Kyra's ending balance at the end of May?

A) $52.54
B) $689.98
C) $742.52
D) $827.27

GO ON TO THE NEXT PAGE

15.

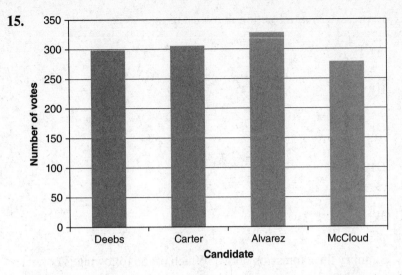

The graph above shows the votes earned by four candidates in a local election.

Each citizen voted for two candidates. About how many citizens voted in all?

A) About 300
B) About 600
C) About 900
D) About 1,200

16. How many millimeters are there in 25 centimeters?

A) 2.5 millimeters
B) 250 millimeters
C) 2,500 millimeters
D) 25,000 millimeters

17. What is the product of 0.12×0.15?

A) 0.0018
B) 0.018
C) 0.18
D) 1.8

18. A scientist studying plant growth collected this set of measurement data: 5 centimeter, 7 centimeter, 7 centimeter, 6 centimeter, x. What is the value of x if the average measurement for the set was 6 centimeter?

A) 4 centimeter
B) 5 centimeter
C) 6 centimeter
D) 7 centimeter

GO ON TO THE NEXT PAGE

19. How would you describe the usual correlation between income and age?

A) None
B) Perfect
C) Positive
D) Negative

20. Which type of graph would best indicate changes in the profits of a corporation over five years' time?

A) Line graph
B) Histogram
C) Circle graph
D) Scatter plot

21. Order this list of numbers from least to greatest.

$$\sqrt{25}, \frac{16}{3}, 4.\overline{98}, 5.01$$

A) $\sqrt{25}, 4.\overline{98}, 5.01, \frac{16}{3}$

B) $4.\overline{98}, \sqrt{25}, \frac{16}{3}, 5.01$

C) $4.\overline{98}, \sqrt{25}, 5.01, \frac{16}{3}$

D) $\frac{16}{3}, 5.01, \sqrt{25}, 4.\overline{98}$

22. A number is two less than the sum of a given number and one.

Which of the following algebraic expressions best represents the statement above?

A) $(n + 1) - 2$
B) $(n + 2) - 1$
C) $n + (2 - 1)$
D) $n = 2 + 1$

23. $|x - 1| = 3$

Which of the following is the solution set for the equation above?

A) $\{4, -4\}$
B) $\{2, -2\}$
C) $\{2, -4\}$
D) $\{-2, 4\}$

24. A botanist is weighing the flowers of several plants in a meadow. Which would be an appropriate unit of measure?

A) Pounds
B) Kilograms
C) Grams
D) Liters

GO ON TO THE NEXT PAGE

25. A plan for a shed is drawn on a 1:10 scale. If the roof of the real shed measures 4 feet by 5 feet, what are the measurements on the plan?

A) 80 inches by 100 inches
B) 40 inches by 50 inches
C) 4.8 inches by 6 inches
D) 4 inches by 5 inches

26. Mrs. Enriquez tipped 22% on her $60 haircut. How much tip did she leave?

A) $5.50
B) $12.00
C) $13.20
D) $14.50

27. Express 85% as a fraction in lowest terms.

A) $\dfrac{17}{20}$

B) $\dfrac{5}{6}$

C) $\dfrac{13}{15}$

D) $\dfrac{9}{10}$

28. Which answer is correct for the product of 0.88×2.1?

A) 0.01848
B) 0.1848
C) 1.848
D) 18.48

GO ON TO THE NEXT PAGE

29.

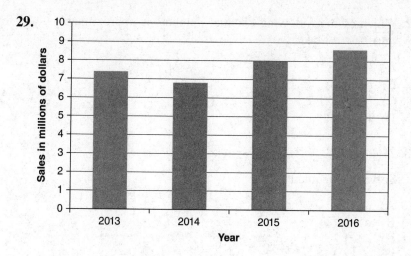

The graph shows the sales at Corporation X over the course of four years.

How much more did Corporation X make in 2016 than in 2015?

A) $6,000
B) $60,000
C) $600,000
D) $6,000,000

30. $1\frac{5}{8} + 1\frac{23}{24}$

Simplify the expression above. Which of the following is correct?

A) $3\frac{19}{24}$

B) $3\frac{7}{12}$

C) $3\frac{5}{16}$

D) $2\frac{5}{24}$

31. Geoff and Angie ordered lunch. Both had a sub at $4.95 apiece, a drink at $1.25 apiece, and chips at $1.35 apiece. Which of the following is a reasonable estimate of the total cost of their lunches?

A) $12
B) $15
C) $20
D) $25

GO ON TO THE NEXT PAGE

32. Which of the following decimal numbers is approximately equal to $\sqrt{50}$?

A) 7.1
B) 7.5
C) 7.9
D) 8.1

33. $2x + 3 > 5$

Solve the inequality.

A) $x > 3$
B) $x > 2$
C) $x > 1$
D) $x \geq 1$

34. Collette collected two dozen eggs in the chicken coop. Of the eggs, 4 were brown, and the rest were white. What was the ratio of brown eggs to white eggs?

A) $\dfrac{1}{6}$

B) $\dfrac{1}{5}$

C) $\dfrac{1}{4}$

D) $\dfrac{1}{3}$

35. A cell phone company charges $0.99 per day and 10 cents per text. If Jacob uses his phone for d days, during which he sends t texts, which expression best illustrates what he spends in d days on his cell plan?

A) $\$0.99d + dt$
B) $\$0.99(d + t)$
C) $\$1.09(dt)$
D) $\$0.99d + \$0.1t$

GO ON TO THE NEXT PAGE

36. $10x - 4x + 4 = 8x - 4$

Which of the following shows the steps to use to solve for x?

A) $6x + 4 = 8x - 4$
$4 = 2x - 4$
$8 = 2x$

B) $6x + (4 - 4) = 8x$
$6x = 8x$

C) $14x - 4x + 4 = -4$
$10x - 4 = -4$
$10x = 0$

D) $10x - 4x = 8x + 8$
$6x = 8x + 8$
$-2x = 8$

STOP. THIS IS THE END OF PART II.

Part III. Science

53 items (47 scored), 63 minutes

1. Which of the following is the function of ribosomes?

A) Respiration
B) Protein synthesis
C) Movement
D) Lipid digestion

2.

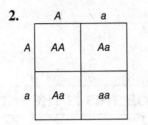

Huntington disease is carried on the dominant allele (A). In this situation, where two heterozygous parents have the disease, what percentage of their offspring are predicted to be disease-free?

A) 0%
B) 25%
C) 50%
D) 100%

3. What does the perimysium surround?

A) The spinal cord
B) The kidneys
C) Bundles of muscles
D) Reproductive organs

4. The elbow is _____ to the shoulder.

Which of the following correctly completes the sentence above?

A) distal
B) cephalic
C) superior
D) anterior

GO ON TO THE NEXT PAGE

5. Which feature of the ear is most medial?

A) Pinna
B) Tympanic membrane
C) Cochlea
D) Outer canal

6. The gallbladder is part of the _____ system.

Which of the following correctly completes the sentence above?

A) endocrine
B) urinary
C) digestive
D) nervous

7. What is the primary hormone secreted by the thyroid gland?

A) Oxytocin
B) TSH
C) Adrenaline
D) T_4

8. Enlargement of the thyroid, commonly known as a goiter, might be expected to affect which of these functions?

A) Swallowing
B) Insulin levels
C) Sleep
D) Digestion

9. Which of the following has the lowest density?

A) Water
B) Cork
C) Aluminum
D) Steel

10. Unlike deductive reasoning, inductive reasoning typically moves from _____ to _____.

Which of the following correctly completes the sentence above?

A) hypothesis; conclusion
B) generalities; specifics
C) observations; hypothesis
D) problem; solution

GO ON TO THE NEXT PAGE

11.

Gas	Carbon Monoxide	Helium	Nitrogen	Oxygen
Molar Mass	28.00 g/mol	4.00 g/mol	14.01 g/mol	16.00 g/mol

Which would you expect to diffuse most rapidly?

A) Carbon monoxide
B) Helium
C) Nitrogen
D) Oxygen

12. What does the diastolic blood pressure number represent?

A) Speed of valve intake and outflow
B) Blood pressure in the veins at rest
C) Pressure in the arteries between heartbeats
D) Force of blood through the arteries with each heartbeat

13.

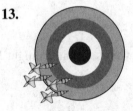

How would you describe the dart throwing indicated?

A) Accurate but not precise
B) Precise but not accurate
C) Both accurate and precise
D) Neither accurate nor precise

14. A student was asked to count birds in a given location over a 24-hour period. Her data would be most valid if she counted

A) birds at one feeder every 6 hours.
B) birds at three feeders at noon and 6:00 P.M.
C) birds at one feeder at noon and 6:00 P.M.
D) birds at three feeders every 6 hours.

GO ON TO THE NEXT PAGE

15. Where does the digestion of carbohydrates begin?

    A) In the mouth
    B) In the stomach
    C) In the pancreas
    D) In the small intestine

16. Which of the following might be an effect of a lower esophageal sphincter that fails to close properly?

    A) Peptic ulcer
    B) Acid reflux
    C) Diverticulitis
    D) Colic

17. Which tool would most likely *not* be part of a quantitative investigation?

    A) Anemometer
    B) Triple beam balance
    C) Calculator
    D) Binoculars

18.

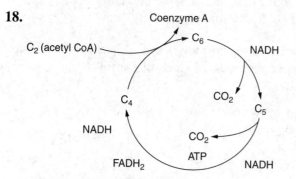

What does this diagram show?

    A) The hydrologic cycle
    B) Active transport
    C) Fermentation
    D) The Krebs cycle

GO ON TO THE NEXT PAGE

19. Is a "balanced diet" the same for all people?

A) Yes, all people should eat the same amounts from the basic food groups.
B) No, the amounts of foods from each food group may vary due to age or sex.
C) No, a "balanced diet" in one part of the world is different from that in another.
D) No, some people can omit a single food group with no ill effects.

20. Which aspect of anorexia may lead to kidney stones?

A) Vitamin deficiency
B) Muscle atrophy
C) Dehydration
D) Swelling and edema

21. Standard temperature and pressure (STP) refers to what conditions?

A) A temperature of 0°C and pressure of 1 atm
B) A temperature of 0 K and pressure of 1 atm
C) A temperature of 273 K and pressure of 0 atm
D) A temperature of 273°C and pressure of 0 atm

22. During an experiment, a scientist uses a spreadsheet to record temperatures. This action corresponds to which of the following steps in the scientific method?

A) Formulating a hypothesis
B) Collecting data
C) Analyzing data
D) Drawing a conclusion

GO ON TO THE NEXT PAGE

23.

PERIODIC TABLE OF THE ELEMENTS

1 H																	2 He
3 Li	4 Be											5 B	6 C	7 N	8 O	9 F	10 Ne
11 Na	12 Mg											13 Al	14 Si	15 P	16 S	17 Ci	18 Ar
19 K	20 Ca	21 Sc	22 Ti	23 V	24 Cr	25 Mn	26 Fe	27 Co	28 Ni	29 Cu	30 Zn	31 Ga	32 Ge	33 As	34 Se	35 Br	36 Kr
37 Rb	38 Sr	39 Y	40 Z	41 Nb	42 Mo	43 Tc	44 Ru	45 Rh	46 Pd	47 Ag	48 Cd	49 In	50 Sn	51 Sb	52 Te	53 I	54 Xe
55 Cs	56 Ba	see below	72 Hf	73 Ta	74 W	75 Re	76 Os	77 It	78 Pt	79 Au	80 Hg	81 Ti	82 Pb	83 Bi	84 Po	85 At	86 Rn
87 Fr	88 Ra	see below	104 Rf	105 Db	106 Sg	107 Bh	108 Hs	109 Mt	110 Ds	111 Rg	112 Uub	113 Uut	114 Uuq	115 Uup	116 Uuh	117 Uus	118 Uuo

■ = Alkali Metals   ▒ = Halogens   ░ = Noble Gases

RARE EARTH ELEMENTS

Lanthanides	57 La	58 Ce	59 Pr	60 Nd	61 Pm	62 Sm	63 Eu	64 Gd	65 Tb	66 Dy	67 Ho	68 Er	69 Tm	70 Yb	71 Lu
Actinides	89 Ac	90 Th	91 Pa	92 U	93 Np	94 Pu	95 Am	96 Cm	97 Bk	98 Cf	99 Es	100 Fm	101 Md	102 No	103 Lr

Where are atoms with the largest atomic radii located?

A) At the top of their group
B) In the middle of their group
C) At the bottom of their group
D) Along the right-hand side

GO ON TO THE NEXT PAGE

24. In which of these glands is growth hormone produced?

    A) Pancreas
    B) Pituitary
    C) Thyroid
    D) Pineal

25. Where would a plantar reflex take place?

    A) In the ankle
    B) In the knee
    C) In the foot
    D) In the jaw

26. Which of these muscles helps rotate the thigh laterally?

    A) Gluteus maximus
    B) Vastus intermedius
    C) Tibialis anterior
    D) Adductor longus

27. How does the circulatory system work with the urinary system?

    A) The circulatory system controls the function of the ureter.
    B) The circulatory system dilutes toxins from the urinary tract.
    C) The kidneys secrete hormones that influence blood flow.
    D) The urinary system removes excess fluid and cleans the blood of waste.

28. In an experiment conducted to compare the life spans of various chicken breeds, the age of each chicken at death is which type of variable?

    A) Dependent
    B) Independent
    C) Controlled
    D) Random

29. One organ system that prevents water loss is the _____ system.

    Which of the following correctly completes the sentence above?

    A) nervous
    B) integumentary
    C) lymphatic
    D) skeletal

GO ON TO THE NEXT PAGE

30. Which of the following bones is part of the axial skeleton?

A) Sternum
B) Pelvis
C) Tibia
D) Femur

31. If the force on an object is doubled, how does its acceleration change?

A) It remains the same.
B) It is halved.
C) It is doubled.
D) It is eliminated.

32. A 2,000-kg car travels at 15 m/s. For a 1,500-kg car traveling at 15 m/s to generate the same momentum, which would need to happen?

A) It would need to accelerate to 20 m/s.
B) It would need to add 500 kg in mass.
C) Both A and B
D) Either A or B

33. Which of the following valves allows blood to flow from the left atrium to the left ventricle?

A) Mitral valve
B) Aortic valve
C) Tricuspid valve
D) Pulmonary valve

34. A scientist's graph of the correlation between the number of cavities in children's teeth and their intake of soda revealed that children who drank the most soda had the most cavities, and children who drank no soda often had no cavities at all. How would you describe this correlation?

A) Scattered
B) Inverse
C) Direct
D) Logarithmic

GO ON TO THE NEXT PAGE

35. Which of the following typically results from plaque buildup in the arteries?

A) Arrhythmia
B) Pericarditis
C) Atherosclerosis
D) Marfan syndrome

36.

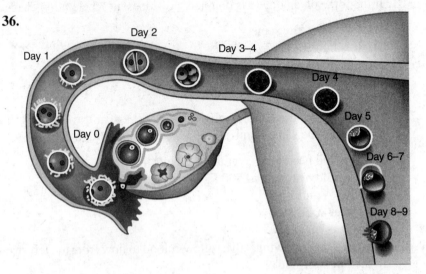

Day 1
Day 2
Day 3–4
Day 4
Day 5
Day 6–7
Day 8–9
Day 0

What does this diagram show?

A) Lactation
B) Meiosis
C) Ovulation
D) Peristalsis

37. What is one danger of drinking juice instead of water?

A) Reduction of metabolic rate
B) Increased retention of fluids
C) Addition of calories to the diet
D) Suppression of hunger

38. For the average person, caloric intake should

A) increase with age after age 25.
B) decline with age after age 25.
C) remain constant over a lifetime.
D) decline, then increase with age.

GO ON TO THE NEXT PAGE

39. You drop a 50-gram metal cube into a cylinder of water. How can you use displacement to find the density of the cube?

A) Measure the volume of the displaced water and divide that into 50.

B) Measure the volume of the displaced water and divide it by 50.

C) Measure the mass of the displaced water and multiply it by 50.

D) Measure the mass of the displaced water and divide it by 50.

40. If you use an eggbeater to beat an egg rapidly for two minutes, what will happen to the temperature of the egg?

A) It will remain constant.

B) It will decline slightly.

C) It will increase slightly.

D) It will decline and then increase.

41. A chemist takes 100 ml of a 0.40 M NaCl solution. She then dilutes it to 1 L. What is the concentration (molarity) of the new solution?

A) 0.04 M NaCl

B) 0.25 M NaCl

C) 0.40 M NaCl

D) 2.5 M NaCl

42. A 10-L tank of oxygen under a pressure of 50 atm would require what pressure to decrease the volume to 1 L?

A) 0.20 atm

B) 20 atm

C) 50 atm

D) 500 atm

43. Which of the following enzymes is found in saliva?

A) Maltase

B) Pepsin

C) Amylase

D) Lactase

GO ON TO THE NEXT PAGE

44.

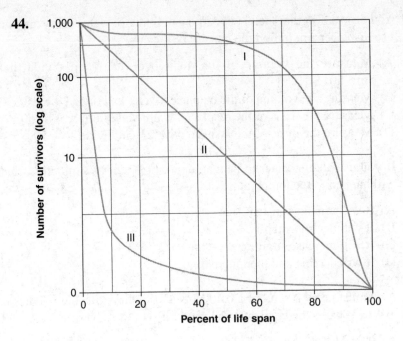

Which survivorship curve indicates the life span of most plants?

A) I
B) II
C) III
D) None of the above

45. Which of the following might be detected by a proprioceptor?

A) Hunger
B) Vibrations
C) Bright light
D) Position in space

46. Which of the following is *not* an endocrine disorder?

A) Diabetes
B) Addison's disease
C) Epstein-Barr disease
D) Cushing's syndrome

47. Which part of the ear is made of cartilage?

A) Incus
B) Auricle
C) Stapes
D) Cochlea

GO ON TO THE NEXT PAGE

48. What is the function of the vacuole?

A) Storage
B) Transport
C) Energy production
D) Mitosis

49. What results from the first stage of meiosis?

A) Two haploid cells
B) Four haploid cells
C) Two diploid cells
D) Four diploid cells

50. In the first stage of respiration, _____, a six-carbon _____ is split in two.

Which of the following correctly completes the sentence above?

A) the Krebs cycle; polypeptide
B) electron transport; molecule of ATP
C) glycolysis; sugar
D) fermentation; chloroplast

51. Which of the following is an example of a ball-and-socket joint?

A) Wrist
B) Thumb
C) Elbow
D) Hip

52. Which of these actions is controlled by skeletal muscles?

A) Eye movement
B) Constriction of blood vessels
C) Heartbeat
D) Dilation of pupils

53. What is the function of B cells?

A) Prevention of virus replication
B) Production of antibodies
C) Repair of damaged tissues
D) Guidance of white blood cells

STOP. THIS IS THE END OF PART III.

Part IV. English and Language Usage

28 items (24 scored), 28 minutes

1. The chemicals in plastic containers may be deleterious to children's health.

   What is the simple subject of this sentence?

   A) children's health
   B) chemicals
   C) plastic
   D) containers

2. Which sentence is written correctly?

   A) Having finished the exam early Rudy checked it over for errors.
   B) Having finished the exam early Rudy checked, it over for errors.
   C) Having finished the exam early, Rudy checked it over for errors.
   D) Having finished, the exam early, Rudy checked it over for errors.

3. The geese were flying south. Hikers were on the mountain. The geese were in a V formation. Hikers spotted the geese.

   To improve sentence fluency, how could you best state the information above in a single sentence?

   A) The geese were flying south in a V formation with hikers on the mountain spotting them.
   B) As the geese flew south, hikers were on the mountain, spotting the geese in a V formation.
   C) Hikers on the mountain spotted geese flying south in a V formation.
   D) In a V formation, geese flying south spotted hikers on the mountain.

4. As the concert concluded, a disorderly ruckus developed at the stadium's easternmost exit.

   Which word in the sentence is a colloquialism?

   A) concluded
   B) disorderly
   C) ruckus
   D) easternmost

GO ON TO THE NEXT PAGE

5. In which stage of the writing process would you most likely remove repetitive information?

A) Revision
B) Planning
C) Citation
D) Drafting

6. Based on the prefix, what does an *andrologist* study?

A) Death and dying
B) Limbs and joints
C) Blood vessels
D) Men's health

7. Only one of the students _____ completed the course.

Which of the following correctly completes the sentence above?

A) have
B) has
C) are
D) is

8. Has anyone here perused Professor Kelso's article on fight-or-flight responses?

What kind of sentence is this?

A) Imperative
B) Interrogative
C) Exclamatory
D) Declarative

9. Dr. Johnson had a serious look when he _____.

Which of the following correctly completes the sentence above?

A) spoke to the patient's parents
B) is speaking to the patient's parents
C) will spcak to the patient's parents
D) has spoken to the patient's parents

GO ON TO THE NEXT PAGE

10. Does your grimace infer that you loathed the performance?

What is the error in this sentence?

A) grimace
B) infer
C) loathed
D) performance

11. Finding the conduit out of the ravine before dusk was both propitious and lucky; in an hour we'd have been trapped by the deluge until daybreak.

Which words are redundant in the sentence above?

A) conduit, deluge
B) dusk, daybreak
C) ravine, deluge
D) propitious, lucky

12. Which sentence is the clearest?

A) I saw the criminals who were arrested watching the TV news.
B) I saw the criminals watching the TV news who were arrested.
C) Watching the TV news, the criminals who were arrested were seen by me.
D) Watching the TV news, I saw the criminals who were arrested.

13. At a presentation he informed us about the dangers of drugs and alcohol in the auditorium.

Which phrase or clause is misplaced in the sentence above?

A) At a presentation
B) about the dangers
C) of drugs and alcohol
D) in the auditorium

14. In which of the following sentences does *conduct* mean "transmit"?

A) Will he conduct his new composition at Sunday's performance?
B) A pair of guides conduct the tourists through the catacombs.
C) The academy students conduct themselves with decorum.
D) Which metal works better to conduct heat, copper or iron?

GO ON TO THE NEXT PAGE

15. We found the movie clumsy, bland, and insipid; the actors, writers, and director seemed to be either fatigued or contemptuous of the audience.

Which words are redundant in the sentence above?

A) clumsy, bland
B) bland, insipid
C) actors, writers
D) fatigued, contemptuous

16. Which of the following is an example of a correctly punctuated sentence?

A) My brother is older than I; nevertheless I often take care of him it seems.
B) My brother is older than I, nevertheless, I often take care of him, it seems.
C) My brother is older than I; nevertheless, I often take care of him, it seems.
D) My brother is older than I; nevertheless I often take care of him, it seems.

17. Which of the following is the best definition of the word *microhabitat*?

A) Great location
B) Meaningless routine
C) Small territory
D) Short garment

18. Which of the following is an example of a simple sentence?

A) The puppy had been warned to stay back but could not help following me down the driveway.
B) The puppy had been warned to stay back; nevertheless, it followed me down the driveway.
C) Although I had warned the puppy to stay back, it followed me down the driveway.
D) I warned the puppy to stay back, but it could not keep from following me down the driveway.

19. Apply a thin film of cream to the affected area once or twice a day depending on the <u>acuteness</u> of the condition.

Which of the following is the meaning of the underlined word above?

A) appeal
B) likelihood
C) stage
D) severity

GO ON TO THE NEXT PAGE

20. Which of the following nouns is written in the correct plural form?

   A) quizes
   B) runner-ups
   C) tomatos
   D) wharves

21. Which of the following is an example of first-person point of view?

   A) Never express yourself in writing unless you want others to read it.
   B) She was unable to answer because her mouth was full.
   C) It was difficult for me to understand exactly what he meant.
   D) Carl and Molly rode the streetcar from Albee Avenue south.

22. Without her handbag, Aunt Julie was practically powerless.

   The word *powerless* serves as which of the following parts of speech in the sentence above?

   A) Noun
   B) Verb
   C) Adjective
   D) Adverb

23. Which of the following sentences has correct subject-verb agreement?

   A) Several of us plans to attend the conference in May.
   B) Some of his writing are just about incomprehensible.
   C) None of those cookies has cooled off enough to eat.
   D) Neither of the candidates speaks particularly well.

24. After many years, the author's work was recognized and acclaimed.

   Which of the following changes the sentence above so that it is written in the active rather than in the passive voice?

   A) The author's work was recognized and acclaimed after many years.
   B) After many years, work by the author was recognized and acclaimed.
   C) After many years, people recognized and acclaimed the author's work.
   D) Work by the author, after many years, was recognized and acclaimed.

25. Which of the following words is written correctly?

   A) long-winded
   B) line-of-fire
   C) length-wise
   D) light-house

GO ON TO THE NEXT PAGE

26. Please have the clients leave _____ umbrellas in the stand over _____.

Which of the following sets of words should be used to fill in the blanks in the sentence above?

A) their; there
B) there; their
C) they're; their
D) their; they're

27. Chloë rarely eats at home anymore _____ she prefers picking up something from the vendor near the library.

Which of the following punctuation marks correctly completes the sentence above?

A) ;
B) :
C) -
D) ,

28. Very few people I know like <u>okra</u>; _____ is apparently an acquired taste.

Which of the following options correctly completes the sentence? The antecedent of the pronoun to be added is underlined.

A) he
B) it
C) them
D) I

STOP. THIS IS THE END OF TEAS PRACTICE TEST 3.

TEAS Practice Test 3: Answer Key

PART I: READING

1. D	19. B	37. A
2. C	20. B	38. C
3. B	21. B	39. A
4. B	22. D	40. D
5. A	23. C	41. B
6. A	24. C	42. D
7. A	25. C	43. A
8. D	26. C	44. C
9. B	27. A	45. B
10. D	28. B	46. D
11. B	29. A	47. A
12. A	30. C	48. B
13. D	31. B	49. D
14. B	32. A	50. B
15. B	33. B	51. B
16. B	34. B	52. C
17. A	35. A	53. C
18. B	36. A	

PART II: MATHEMATICS

1. A	13. B	25. C
2. D	14. C	26. C
3. C	15. B	27. A
4. B	16. B	28. C
5. A	17. B	29. C
6. B	18. B	30. B
7. D	19. C	31. B
8. C	20. A	32. A
9. C	21. C	33. C
10. A	22. A	34. B
11. A	23. D	35. D
12. D	24. C	36. A

PART III: SCIENCE

1. B	19. B	37. C
2. B	20. C	38. B
3. C	21. A	39. A
4. A	22. B	40. C
5. C	23. C	41. A
6. C	24. B	42. D
7. D	25. C	43. C
8. A	26. A	44. C
9. B	27. D	45. D
10. C	28. A	46. C
11. B	29. B	47. B
12. C	30. A	48. A
13. B	31. C	49. C
14. D	32. D	50. C
15. A	33. A	51. D
16. B	34. C	52. A
17. D	35. C	53. B
18. D	36. C	

PART IV: ENGLISH AND LANGUAGE USAGE

1. B	11. D	21. C
2. C	12. D	22. C
3. C	13. D	23. D
4. C	14. D	24. C
5. A	15. B	25. A
6. D	16. C	26. A
7. B	17. C	27. A
8. B	18. A	28. B
9. A	19. D	
10. B	20. D	

TEAS Practice Test 3: Explanatory Answers

Part I: Reading

1. (D) Jealousy is an emotion felt by one sister toward the other. It is an underlying theme of the story.

2. (C) Like most works of fiction, this story is written primarily to entertain the reader.

3. (B) Teresa holds the dress up and imagines wearing it. It is reasonable to assume that she wants it for herself.

4. (B) Only choice B is something that did not actually happen. It is Teresa's belief, not a fact.

5. (A) The differences between the girls are clearly described in the first paragraph, making choices B and C incorrect. Despite these differences, the sisters treat each other kindly, making choice D incorrect.

6. (A) Narrative writing tells a story.

7. (A) The topic sentence explains what the remaining material will be about.

8. (D) The writer does not compare termites to other creatures (choice A), does not tell readers to stop killing termites (choice B), and does not tell a story at all (choice C). She points out potential good sides of a destructive insect, making choice D the only possible answer.

9. (B) The description of termite consumption is presented in a matter-of-fact tone, making choices C and D unlikely. The writer says, "They are said to have a nutty taste and to be rich in protein," which indicates that she has not tasted them herself (choice A). Only choice B fits here.

10. (D) Expository writing is designed to explain or inform.

11. (B) The writer is not biased toward or against termites (choices A and D), and she certainly does not approve of termites' destructive habits (choice C). She can see good as well as bad in the insects, making choice B the correct answer.

12. (A) The final paragraph begins with a statement of opinion ("Termites are important in other ways") and goes on to list examples that support that opinion.

13. (D) Determine which phrase makes sense in the context of the paragraph. In this case, the FDA may conduct its own review or inspection to determine the effectiveness of a recall.

14. (B) In a recall, the product in question is pulled from the shelves of retailers.

15. (B) *Eleanor Roosevelt* might be the topic, but the main idea is that she was more than just a first lady.

16. (B) Although the writer does show a bias toward the subject (choice C), the main purpose of the paragraph is to tell what Roosevelt did to earn the writer's approval.

17. (A) The list of ingredients includes wheat, which is harmful to those with a gluten allergy.

18. (B) The list of ingredients should indicate that the product is some kind of sauce.

19. (B) The darkest bar is the birth weight. The shortest of those dark bars is the one for child A, coming in at not quite halfway between 2 and 3 kilograms.

20. (B) The medium-colored bar is the one for 2 months. The tallest of those bars is between 5 and 5.5 kilograms. The shortest is between 3.5 and 4 kilograms. The difference is greater than 1 but less than 2.

21. (B) It may be easiest to visualize this if you actually draw a picture.

blue	white	blue red	white	blue	white red	blue	white	blue red	white	blue	white red

Four sections remain white.

22. (D) A glossary of terms contains definitions of words in a text.

23. (C) One kilogram = 2.2 pounds. Since kilograms are greater than pounds, kilograms must be the inner ring of numbers on this scale, and pounds must be the outer ring. Therefore, 9 pounds is about equal to 4 kilograms.

24. (C) The writer remarks that "there is no such thing as too much protection." She clearly thinks the rules are reasonable.

25. (C) *Overkill* is used to refer to the rules in terms of their excessive harshness.

26. (C) "Formation of" lymph is first discussed on page 139.

27. (A) The family will spend 9:30 to 10:30 in one part of the zoo, 10:30 to 11:30 in a second, 11:30 to 12:30 in a part of the zoo that contains food, and 12:30 to 1:30 in a fourth part of the zoo. The only list that has a third section with food is choice A.

28. (B) If they move clockwise, they will visit Wild Asia, Wild Oceans, Wild Africa, and Wild Americas, in that order. Wild Americas has a gift shop.

29. (A) This short description of a graduation makes sense when ordered (C), (D), (B), (A). The final action is James's movement offstage with his diploma.

30. (C) Items A to E must all fit within the category of "Types of Lesions." On the list of choices, only cysts (choice C) are types of lesions.

31. (B) Working step by step: *demon, wemon, women, enwom, entom, entomb.*

32. (A) An appeal to voters is often published on the editorial page as a letter to the editor.

33. (B) Predators are carnivores, not herbivores.

34. (B) Written materials and artifacts from the time in question can be primary sources, whereas a work such as a biography that is written after the event may draw from multiple primary sources but is considered a secondary source.

35. (A) A recent travel guide would contain a list of places to stay.

36. (A) Even if you never saw the word before, you should be able to determine the meaning from the sentence context.

37. (A) All of the choices are possible reasons to use italics in text, but only choice A seems to fit—the writer wants to stress the word.

38. (C) Only mercury is identified as a metal (choice A), and only alcohol is dyed (choice B). Unlike mercury, alcohol does not have toxic fumes (choice D). The best answer is choice C.

39. (A) The pulse rate is indicated next to the abbreviation *PUL.*

40. (D) You do not need to do as much computation here as you may think. Even at 8 percent, no product will have a sales tax greater than $2. The tax on Shorebird's item brings it over $25, meaning that there is no shipping cost.

41. (B) For "Sign Language," the yellow page tells you to turn to "Translators and Interpreters."

42. (D) Krystal's ad says that the salon is open "Mon–Sat."

43. (A) Each bottle contains 60 geltabs. The first bottle costs around $16, and the second is half-price, or around $8.

44. (C) The second half of the sentence should help you decipher the meaning of the word.

45. (B) The inspector states that he has called the family together to reveal the identity and motive of the thief, or his interpretation of a crime.

46. (D) The scene is typical of certain types of detective novels.

47. (A) The reader may need to look under *P* for *plover* rather than *S* for *semipalmated*, but he should certainly start with the index.

48. (B) In problems of this kind, it may help to draw a picture. You start with five pairs of socks, in brown, black, green, blue, and red. After step 2, you have four pairs of socks and one single green sock. After step 3, you have three pairs of socks, one single green sock, and one single red sock. After step 4, you have two pairs of socks, one single green sock, and one single red sock. After step 5, you have two pairs of socks, two additional pairs of green socks, and one single red sock, for four pairs in all.

49. (D) The e-mail identifies Abbey as the charter school. According to the graph, Abbey School had a population of 325 in the year 2010.

50. (B) The e-mail seems to indicate that reduction in housing along the waterfront may be the cause of reduced population in Abbey School. The only logical question to ask is choice B—did a substantial number of children from those now-vanished apartments attend Abbey School? If not, the reason for the loss of population must be something else.

51. (B) The News History Gallery contains "newspapers from the early days of publishing," so a paper from the 18th century is likely to be included.

52. (C) Most people "view the museum from the top down," and the top floor has a "fabulous view."

53. (C) The author makes a recommendation in the opening paragraph, saying that the museum "is worth a visit both for its stunning exhibits and for its fascinating interactive displays." The other answer choices may be true, but they are not specifically given as reasons for the recommendation.

Part II: Mathematics

1. (A) To add mixed numbers, first express them as improper fractions. In this case, $4\frac{2}{3}$ may be expressed as $\frac{14}{3}$, and $6\frac{1}{2}$ may be expressed as $\frac{13}{2}$. Next, find the common denominator—6. $\frac{14}{3} = \frac{28}{6}$, and $\frac{13}{2} = \frac{39}{6}$. Add the numerators: $28 + 39 = 67$. $\frac{67}{6} = 11\frac{1}{6}$.

2. (D) The brand-name arthritis drug costs 135×12 for a year, or \$1,620. The generic arthritis drug costs 30×12 for a year, or \$360. Subtract to find the difference: $1,620 - 360 = 1,260$. Another way to solve this is to find the difference for a month: $135 - 30 = 105$. Then multiply by 12 months: $105 \times 12 = 1,260$.

3. (C) Simply read across to find the totals: The hospital had 85 staff members in 2014 and 75 in 2016. $85 - 75 = 10$.

4. (B) The area of the rectangle is 3 cm $\times$ 7 cm, or 21 cm^2. The area of the triangle is $\frac{1}{2}$ base $\times$ height, or $\frac{1}{2}(3 \times 2)$. Adding 3 cm^2 + 21 cm^2 = 24 cm^2.

5. (A) Start by multiplying the squares: $4x \times 4x = 16x^2$. Now multiply $4x \times -1$ and $4x \times 1$, for $-4x + 4x$, or 0 in all. Finally, multiply the final digits: -1×1, equaling -1. The solution is $16x^2 - 1$.

6. (B) Think: $0.80x = 24$. Solve: $x = 24 \div 0.80$. The answer is 30.

7. (D) Set this up as a proportion: $\frac{2}{5} = \frac{x}{145}$. You may cross-multiply to solve: $2 \times 145 = 5x$. $290 = 5x$. $x = \frac{290}{5}$, or 58.

8. (C) If 1 mile equals 1.6 kilometers, 12 miles equals 1.6×12, or 19.2 kilometers.

9. (C) Multiplying a number with two digits to the right of the decimal point by a number with one digit to the right of the decimal point should result in a product with three digits to the right of the decimal point. However, since the final digit is 0, you can state the product as 0.33 rather than 0.330.

10. (A) First, determine how much Stu spent for the cups: $0.25 × 6 = $1.50. Then find out what he spent for the plates: $0.75 × 6 = $4.50. Add those sums: $1.50 + $4.50 = $6.00. Finally, subtract that total from $10.00: $10.00 − $6.00 = $4.00.

11. (A) The mode is the most frequent score.

12. (D) 1.25 equals $1\dfrac{25}{100}$, or $1\dfrac{1}{4}$ in lowest terms.

13. (B) Begin by expressing the mixed numbers as improper fractions: $3\dfrac{1}{2} = \dfrac{7}{2}$, and $1\dfrac{1}{10} = \dfrac{11}{10}$. To divide by a fraction, multiply by its reciprocal. Therefore, $\dfrac{7}{2} \div \dfrac{11}{10} = \dfrac{7}{2} \times \dfrac{10}{11}$, or $\dfrac{70}{22}$. Now reduce to lowest terms: $\dfrac{70}{22} \div \dfrac{2}{2} = \dfrac{35}{11}$. Finally, express $\dfrac{35}{11}$ as a mixed number: $3\dfrac{2}{11}$.

14. (C) Start by adding Kyra's opening balance to her deposit to find how much she had before she began to withdraw funds: $689.98 + $1,027.29 = $1,717.27. Now add up the withdrawals: $40 + $40 + $770 + $40 + $84.75 = $974.75. Finally, subtract the withdrawals from the amount in the account: $1,717.27 − $974.75 = $742.52.

15. (B) If each voter voted for two candidates, the total voters must equal $\dfrac{1}{2}$ the total votes. Since a quick estimate of the total votes equals about 300 × 4, or 1,200, the number of voters must be around 600.

16. (B) One centimeter = 10 millimeters, so 25 centimeters = 250 millimeters.

17. (B) Multiplying two numbers with two digits to the right of the decimal point should result in a product with four digits to the right of the decimal point. However, in this case, the final digit, 0, is dropped off.

18. (B) If the average is 6 cm, then (5 cm + 7 cm + 7 cm + 6 cm + x) ÷ 5 = 6 cm. Do the addition: (25 cm + x) ÷ 5 = 6 cm. It should be easy to see that the answer that makes the equation true is 5 cm.

19. (C) Typically, older workers make more money than their younger associates, meaning that age and income rise in the same direction, creating a positive correlation. However, because income does not rise in a fixed proportion compared to age, the correlation is not perfect (choice B).

20. (A) A line graph is designed to show change over time.

21. (C) The square root of 25 is 5, and $\dfrac{16}{3} = 5.333....$

22. (A) If n = the given number, the sum of that number and 1 is $n + 1$. To find the number that is 2 less, subtract 2 from $(n + 1)$.

23. (D) The bars mean "absolute value," which denotes the distance from zero on the number line and is always expressed as a positive number. $4 - 1 = 3$, so one of the numbers is 4. In addition, $-2 - 1 = -3$, and the absolute value of -3 is 3.

24. (C) Flowers don't weigh much, so grams would be a better unit than pounds or kilograms. Liters measure liquids.

25. (C) You can find the answer by setting up a proportion. First convert the feet to inches: 4 feet = 48 inches. Then solve the proportion: $\frac{1}{10} = \frac{x}{48}$, so $x = 4.8$ inches. You do not even need to complete the proportion for 5 feet, or 60 inches.

26. (C) Solve by multiplying $60 by 22%, or 0.22: $60 \times 0.22 = \$13.20$.

27. (A) $85\% = \frac{85}{100}. \ \frac{85}{100} \div \frac{5}{5} = \frac{17}{20}.$

28. (C) Try estimating. The numbers being multiplied are a little less than 1 and a little more than 2, so the answer will be around 2. You can find the answer without working out the computation.

29. (C) The company made around $8 million in 2015, and a little less than $9 million in 2016, so the best answer must be choice C.

30. (B) Express the mixed numbers as improper fractions: $\frac{13}{8} + \frac{47}{24}$. Then find the lowest common denominator and give both fractions the same denominator: $\frac{39}{24} + \frac{47}{24} = \frac{86}{24}$. Finally, express the fraction as a mixed number: $3\frac{14}{24}$, and express that in lowest terms: $3\frac{7}{12}$.

31. (B) Rounding the numbers to the nearest dollar can help you estimate fairly accurately: $5 + \$5 + \$1 + \$1 + \$1 + \$1 = \$14$. The closest answer is choice B.

32. (A) You know that the square root of 49 is 7, so the square root of 50 must be close to 7. $8^2 = 64$, which is 15 more than 49, so a square of 7.5 is likely to be closer to 56 or 57 than to 50. The best estimate is choice A.

33. (C) You may solve this by trial and error, or you may work it out algebraically: $2x + 3 > 5$; $2x > 2$, so $x > 1$.

34. (B) Collette collected 24 eggs in all. Of those, 4 were brown, and 20 must have been white. The ratio is 4:20, or, in lowest terms, $\frac{1}{5}$.

35. (D) $\$0.99d$ represents the total cost of the cell phone, and $\$0.10t$ or $\$0.1t$ represents the total cost of texting. Adding the two gives you the total cost for d days. For example, if Jacob uses the phone for 30 days, sending 50 texts in that time, he will spend $\$0.99(30) + \$0.1(50) = \$29.70 + \$5.00$, or $\$34.70$.

36. (A) Do the easiest addition/subtraction first: $10x - 4x = 6x$. Subtracting $6x$ from both sides of the equation gives you 4 on one side and $2x - 4$ on the other. Adding 4 to each side gives you $8 = 2x$, meaning that $x = 4$. Plug that back into the original equation to check:

$$10(4) - 4(4) + 4 = 8(4) - 4$$
$$40 - 16 + 4 = 32 - 4$$
$$24 + 4 = 28$$

Part III: Science

1. (B) Ribosomes decode RNA and link amino acids to form the polypeptide chains that make up proteins in the process known as translation.

2. (B) If the disease is carried on the dominant allele, only the *aa* combination of recessive genes represents a disease-free offspring.

3. (C) The perimysium is a covering of connective tissue that surrounds a bundle of skeletal muscle fibers, or fascicle.

4. (A) If you extend your arms, the elbow is further from the torso than the shoulder is, making it more distal.

5. (C) The most medial feature is the one closest to the middle of the body.

6. (C) The gallbladder stores the fat-digesting bile produced by the liver.

7. (D) Thyroxine (T_4) aids in the regulation of metabolism.

8. (A) A goiter may put pressure on the trachea and esophagus, causing difficulty in breathing or swallowing.

9. (B) Cork has holes throughout that reduce the volume of matter present (the cork is replaced by air), making it less dense than many other materials.

10. (C) In inductive reasoning, a hypothesis follows from a series of observations.

11. (B) A gas with low molar mass will diffuse more rapidly than one with greater molar mass.

12. (C) Blood pressure is reported as systolic over diastolic numbers. The systolic number is the pressure on the arteries as the heart pumps (choice D). The diastolic number is the pressure as the heart rests between beats (choice C).

13. (B) The dart throws were precise, in that they corresponded closely with one another. However, since they missed the center of the target, they were not accurate.

14. (D) The more measurements made, the more valid the data are likely to be. Using three sites rather than one allows the researcher to increase observations.

15. (A) Digestion of carbohydrates begins in the mouth, where salivary glands secrete salivary amylase, which starts to break down the polysaccharides in food into maltose, a disaccharide formed from two units of glucose.

16. (B) When the ring of muscle that separates the esophagus from the stomach fails to close properly, stomach acid may move up into the esophagus, causing the recurring heartburn known as acid reflux disease.

17. (D) Choices A, B, and C are definitely quantitative, in that they provide specific measurements, but choice D may or may not be.

18. (D) The Krebs cycle is part of the second step in the production of energy. During the Krebs cycle, the pyruvate molecules produced during glycolysis are converted into ATP.

19. (B) The optimal quantities of each nutrient vary with a person's sex, age, weight, and activity level. For example, very young children need more fat than adults do, and women need more iron-rich and calcium-rich foods than men do.

20. (C) Chronic dehydration due to fasting and overuse of laxatives can harm the kidneys in a variety of ways, including the formation of stones.

21. (A) STP corresponds to 273 K (0°C) and 1 atm of pressure.

22. (B) The collection and organization of data is part of the experimental phase of the scientific process.

23. (C) On the periodic table, the atomic radii of atoms tend to decrease across a period from left to right and increase down a group, with the largest radii appearing in group I and at the bottoms of groups.

24. (B) Growth hormone is produced and secreted by the anterior pituitary gland, which also assists in regulating stress, lactation, and reproduction.

25. (C) The plantar reflex takes place when the sole of the foot is stroked. Normally, the toes flex downward. If they flex upward in adults, in what is known as the Babinski response, this may be indicative of nerve damage or disease.

26. (A) The gluteus maximus is one of several muscles that help rotate the thigh; others include the piriformus and the gemellus superior. Of the other possible responses, choice B helps extend the leg, choice C flexes the ankle, and choice D flexes and extends the thigh.

27. (D) The urinary system eliminates water, urea, and other waste products from the body in the form of urine.

28. (A) The dependent variable (choice A) is the one that is affected by the independent variable (choice B). In this case, the breed of the subjects is not affected by the age of the subjects.

29. (B) The integumentary system (the skin and its appendages) waterproofs the body from outside and guards against excess fluid loss from inside.

30. (A) The axial skeleton is made up of the vertebral column, the skull, 12 pairs of ribs, and the sternum. Choices B, C, and D are part of the appendicular skeleton.

31. (C) As long as the mass of the object remains the same, the relationship between force and acceleration is direct. Doubling the force will double the acceleration.

32. (D) Momentum is the product of velocity and mass. The first car's momentum is $2,000 \times 15 = 30,000$ kg · m/s. The second car's momentum is $1,500 \times 15 = 22,500$ kg · m/s. For its momentum to equal that of the first car, it could either accelerate to 20 m/s or add 500 kg to its mass.

33. (A) The mitral valve opens to let blood flow from the top left chamber of the heart to the lower left chamber of the heart. Of the other choices, the aortic valve (choice B) lets blood flow from the left ventricle to the aorta, the tricuspid valve (choice C) lets blood flow from the right atrium to the right ventricle, and the pulmonary valve (choice D) lets blood flow from the right ventricle through the pulmonary artery.

34. (C) If large values of one variable match large values of the other, and small values of the first variable match small values of the other, the correlation is direct, whether the values increase or decrease.

35. (C) Atherosclerosis is commonly referred to as "hardening of the arteries." It occurs when cholesterol, fatty substances, calcium, and other materials block blood flow through an artery. Usually, the substances begin to build up due to some sort of damage to the lining of the arterial wall.

36. (C) The diagram shows the discharge of an ovum (oocyte) and its progression through the fallopian tube to the uterus.

37. (C) Juice contains sugar, so that even grapefruit juice has about 93 calories per cup. Water contains no calories at all.

38. (B) The height of calorie intake for healthy, active people is approximately their mid-20s. After that, calorie intake should decline slightly as energy needs decline.

39. (A) Density = mass/volume. Measuring the volume of the displaced water gives you the volume of the cube, and dividing that volume into the mass, 50, gives you the cube's density.

40. (C) Beating the egg rapidly causes its temperature to increase because of the energy released by the work you are doing.

41. (A) The number of moles remains constant, but the volume increases tenfold, so the moles/volume (molarity) is $\frac{1}{10}$ the original.

42. (D) If $p_1V_1 = p_2V_2$, then $10 \text{ L} \times 50 \text{ atm} = 1 \text{ L} \times 500 \text{ atm}$.

43. (C) Amylase is one of a few enzymes that begin the process of digestion in the mouth. It converts starch into simple sugars.

44. (C) Line III indicates a species in which offspring die off in large numbers shortly after birth, and only a few individuals survive for an extended life span. This would be typical of most plants.

45. (D) Sensory receptors may be classified by the location of stimuli. Exteroceptors detect stimuli outside the body, such as vibrations (choice B) or light (choice C). Interoceptors detect stimuli inside the body, such as hunger (choice A). Proprioceptors detect changes in the stretch of the organs they occupy, especially muscles, tendons, and ligaments, and thus provide information on position and posture (choice D).

46. (C) Epstein-Barr is a viral disease. Diabetes (choice A) is a malfunction of the pancreas, Addison's disease (choice B) is a malfunction of the adrenals, and Cushing's syndrome (choice D) is a malfunction of the pituitary.

47. (B) The auricle is the outer section of the ear, the part that is external to the head. It is composed primarily of cartilage. The other three choices are primarily bone—choice A, the incus (anvil), and choice C, the stapes (stirrup), are two of the small bones of the middle ear; and choice D, the cochlea, is a bony spiral in the inner ear.

48. (A) The vacuole may contain water, food, or waste products.

49. (C) In the first stage of meiosis, meoisis I, the parent cell splits into two diploid cells. In the second stage, meiosis II, those two cells split to form four haploid cells, each with only one set of chromosomes from the parent cell.

50. (C) Glycolysis is the breakdown of sugar into pyruvic acid, with ATP as a by-product.

51. (D) The hip (choice D) is a ball-and-socket joint in which the rounded head of the femur rests in the socket formed by the pelvis. Of the other examples, the wrist (choice A) is a condyloid joint (and the carpals of the wrist are gliding joints), the thumb (choice B) is a saddle joint, and the elbow (choice C) is a hinge joint.

52. (A) Eye movement is controlled by skeletal muscles, which contract and relax to manipulate body parts. Constriction of blood vessels (choice B) and dilation of pupils (choice D) are controlled by smooth muscle cells. Heartbeat (choice C) is controlled by cardiac muscles.

53. (B) B cells are lymphocytes that cruise the body seeking invaders. They may mature into plasma cells that produce specific antibodies.

Part IV: English and Language Usage

1. (B) A prepositional phrase intervenes between the subject and verb, which may confuse you. Think: "What may be deleterious?" The answer is the chemicals (choice B), not the containers (choice C).

2. (C) A comma must appear between the introductory phrase *Having finished the exam early* and the independent clause *Rudy checked it over for errors.* No other commas are needed.

3. (C) Reading the choices aloud may help you determine which choice has a logical order of phrases and clauses. The least convoluted sentence is choice C.

4. (C) A ruckus is a noisy fight. The word is informal and colloquial.

5. (A) Revision is the process of editing for sense, organization, and accuracy as well as proofreading for grammar, capitalization, and punctuation.

6. (D) The prefix *andro-* means "man," as in *androgen* or *androgyny*.

7. (B) The subject is *one*, which is singular. Therefore, the correct verb must agree with a singular subject. *Is completed* (choice D) is ungrammatical.

8. (B) An interrogative sentence asks a question.

9. (A) In this type of question, you must make sure that the tense of verbs remains consistent. Because *had* is past tense, the correct answer contains another past-tense verb, *spoke*.

10. (B) To infer is to deduce, or conclude. A person's grimace cannot do that. A grimace may, however, imply or indicate loathing.

11. (D) *Propitious* and *lucky* mean the same thing and are thus redundant, or repetitive.

12. (D) Who was watching the TV news? Was it the criminals, or was it the person speaking? Only choice D places the modifying phrase next to the word it modifies.

13. (D) Look for the phrase that, if moved around, would improve the sentence. The danger of drugs and alcohol is not limited to the auditorium; a better sentence would be "At a presentation in the auditorium, he informed us about the dangers of drugs and alcohol."

14. (D) When used as a verb, *conduct* has a variety of meanings; among them are "to direct" (choice A), "to lead" (choice B), and "to behave" (choice C). In choice D, the word means "to transmit via conduction."

15. (B) Something that is bland and insipid might also be called *unexciting*.

16. (C) The sentence is composed of two independent clauses, calling for a semicolon to divide them. A comma after the transitional word *nevertheless* is traditional, as is the comma before the parenthetical element "it seems."

17. (C) The root *micro*, as in *microscopic,* means "small," and the word *habitat* means "territory."

18. (A) A simple sentence has just one subject and verb. Although sentence A contains the word *but*, it combines two predicates, not two clauses, keeping the sentence simple in construction.

19. (D) *Acute* means "sharp" and may refer to anything that is intense and severe.

20. (D) *Wharf*, like many words that end in *f* or *fe*, becomes plural with a change from *f* to *v*. The correct spelling of the other plurals would be *quizzes, runners-up,* and *tomatoes*.

21. (C) First-person pronouns include *I* and *we*. Choices B and D are in the third person, and choice A is in the second person.

22. (C) *Powerless* modifies *Aunt Julie*, which is a noun. Adjectives modify nouns.

23. (D) Sentence A has a plural subject, *several*. Although *some* may be singular or plural, in sentence B it relates to *writing*, which is singular. Although *none* may be singular or plural, in sentence C it relates to *cookies*, which is plural. The subject *neither* (choice D) is always singular.

24. (C) Active voice expresses an action performed by a subject rather than an action performed on a subject. In this case, you must add a subject, *people*, to create an active sentence.

25. (A) *Lengthwise* (choice C) and *lighthouse* (choice D) are closed compounds, and *line of fire* (choice B) is an open compound that does not take hyphens.

26. (A) *Their* means "belonging to them." *There* means "in that place." *They're* means "they are."

27. (A) The sentence is composed of two independent clauses and must be divided by a semicolon.

28. (B) *Okra* is the antecedent, and the only pronoun that can replace it is *it*.

TEAS PRACTICE TEST 4

TEAS Practice Test 4: Answer Sheet

READING

1 (A) (B) (C) (D)
2 (A) (B) (C) (D)
3 (A) (B) (C) (D)
4 (A) (B) (C) (D)
5 (A) (B) (C) (D)
6 (A) (B) (C) (D)
7 (A) (B) (C) (D)
8 (A) (B) (C) (D)
9 (A) (B) (C) (D)
10 (A) (B) (C) (D)
11 (A) (B) (C) (D)
12 (A) (B) (C) (D)
13 (A) (B) (C) (D)
14 (A) (B) (C) (D)
15 (A) (B) (C) (D)
16 (A) (B) (C) (D)
17 (A) (B) (C) (D)
18 (A) (B) (C) (D)

19 (A) (B) (C) (D)
20 (A) (B) (C) (D)
21 (A) (B) (C) (D)
22 (A) (B) (C) (D)
23 (A) (B) (C) (D)
24 (A) (B) (C) (D)
25 (A) (B) (C) (D)
26 (A) (B) (C) (D)
27 (A) (B) (C) (D)
28 (A) (B) (C) (D)
29 (A) (B) (C) (D)
30 (A) (B) (C) (D)
31 (A) (B) (C) (D)
32 (A) (B) (C) (D)
33 (A) (B) (C) (D)
34 (A) (B) (C) (D)
35 (A) (B) (C) (D)
36 (A) (B) (C) (D)

37 (A) (B) (C) (D)
38 (A) (B) (C) (D)
39 (A) (B) (C) (D)
40 (A) (B) (C) (D)
41 (A) (B) (C) (D)
42 (A) (B) (C) (D)
43 (A) (B) (C) (D)
44 (A) (B) (C) (D)
45 (A) (B) (C) (D)
46 (A) (B) (C) (D)
47 (A) (B) (C) (D)
48 (A) (B) (C) (D)
49 (A) (B) (C) (D)
50 (A) (B) (C) (D)
51 (A) (B) (C) (D)
52 (A) (B) (C) (D)
53 (A) (B) (C) (D)

MATHEMATICS

1 (A) (B) (C) (D)
2 (A) (B) (C) (D)
3 (A) (B) (C) (D)
4 (A) (B) (C) (D)
5 (A) (B) (C) (D)
6 (A) (B) (C) (D)
7 (A) (B) (C) (D)
8 (A) (B) (C) (D)
9 (A) (B) (C) (D)
10 (A) (B) (C) (D)
11 (A) (B) (C) (D)
12 (A) (B) (C) (D)

13 (A) (B) (C) (D)
14 (A) (B) (C) (D)
15 (A) (B) (C) (D)
16 (A) (B) (C) (D)
17 (A) (B) (C) (D)
18 (A) (B) (C) (D)
19 (A) (B) (C) (D)
20 (A) (B) (C) (D)
21 (A) (B) (C) (D)
22 (A) (B) (C) (D)
23 (A) (B) (C) (D)
24 (A) (B) (C) (D)

25 (A) (B) (C) (D)
26 (A) (B) (C) (D)
27 (A) (B) (C) (D)
28 (A) (B) (C) (D)
29 (A) (B) (C) (D)
30 (A) (B) (C) (D)
31 (A) (B) (C) (D)
32 (A) (B) (C) (D)
33 (A) (B) (C) (D)
34 (A) (B) (C) (D)
35 (A) (B) (C) (D)
36 (A) (B) (C) (D)

SCIENCE

1	Ⓐ Ⓑ Ⓒ Ⓓ	19	Ⓐ Ⓑ Ⓒ Ⓓ	37	Ⓐ Ⓑ Ⓒ Ⓓ
2	Ⓐ Ⓑ Ⓒ Ⓓ	20	Ⓐ Ⓑ Ⓒ Ⓓ	38	Ⓐ Ⓑ Ⓒ Ⓓ
3	Ⓐ Ⓑ Ⓒ Ⓓ	21	Ⓐ Ⓑ Ⓒ Ⓓ	39	Ⓐ Ⓑ Ⓒ Ⓓ
4	Ⓐ Ⓑ Ⓒ Ⓓ	22	Ⓐ Ⓑ Ⓒ Ⓓ	40	Ⓐ Ⓑ Ⓒ Ⓓ
5	Ⓐ Ⓑ Ⓒ Ⓓ	23	Ⓐ Ⓑ Ⓒ Ⓓ	41	Ⓐ Ⓑ Ⓒ Ⓓ
6	Ⓐ Ⓑ Ⓒ Ⓓ	24	Ⓐ Ⓑ Ⓒ Ⓓ	42	Ⓐ Ⓑ Ⓒ Ⓓ
7	Ⓐ Ⓑ Ⓒ Ⓓ	25	Ⓐ Ⓑ Ⓒ Ⓓ	43	Ⓐ Ⓑ Ⓒ Ⓓ
8	Ⓐ Ⓑ Ⓒ Ⓓ	26	Ⓐ Ⓑ Ⓒ Ⓓ	44	Ⓐ Ⓑ Ⓒ Ⓓ
9	Ⓐ Ⓑ Ⓒ Ⓓ	27	Ⓐ Ⓑ Ⓒ Ⓓ	45	Ⓐ Ⓑ Ⓒ Ⓓ
10	Ⓐ Ⓑ Ⓒ Ⓓ	28	Ⓐ Ⓑ Ⓒ Ⓓ	46	Ⓐ Ⓑ Ⓒ Ⓓ
11	Ⓐ Ⓑ Ⓒ Ⓓ	29	Ⓐ Ⓑ Ⓒ Ⓓ	47	Ⓐ Ⓑ Ⓒ Ⓓ
12	Ⓐ Ⓑ Ⓒ Ⓓ	30	Ⓐ Ⓑ Ⓒ Ⓓ	48	Ⓐ Ⓑ Ⓒ Ⓓ
13	Ⓐ Ⓑ Ⓒ Ⓓ	31	Ⓐ Ⓑ Ⓒ Ⓓ	49	Ⓐ Ⓑ Ⓒ Ⓓ
14	Ⓐ Ⓑ Ⓒ Ⓓ	32	Ⓐ Ⓑ Ⓒ Ⓓ	50	Ⓐ Ⓑ Ⓒ Ⓓ
15	Ⓐ Ⓑ Ⓒ Ⓓ	33	Ⓐ Ⓑ Ⓒ Ⓓ	51	Ⓐ Ⓑ Ⓒ Ⓓ
16	Ⓐ Ⓑ Ⓒ Ⓓ	34	Ⓐ Ⓑ Ⓒ Ⓓ	52	Ⓐ Ⓑ Ⓒ Ⓓ
17	Ⓐ Ⓑ Ⓒ Ⓓ	35	Ⓐ Ⓑ Ⓒ Ⓓ	53	Ⓐ Ⓑ Ⓒ Ⓓ
18	Ⓐ Ⓑ Ⓒ Ⓓ	36	Ⓐ Ⓑ Ⓒ Ⓓ		

ENGLISH AND LANGUAGE USAGE

1	Ⓐ Ⓑ Ⓒ Ⓓ	11	Ⓐ Ⓑ Ⓒ Ⓓ	21	Ⓐ Ⓑ Ⓒ Ⓓ
2	Ⓐ Ⓑ Ⓒ Ⓓ	12	Ⓐ Ⓑ Ⓒ Ⓓ	22	Ⓐ Ⓑ Ⓒ Ⓓ
3	Ⓐ Ⓑ Ⓒ Ⓓ	13	Ⓐ Ⓑ Ⓒ Ⓓ	23	Ⓐ Ⓑ Ⓒ Ⓓ
4	Ⓐ Ⓑ Ⓒ Ⓓ	14	Ⓐ Ⓑ Ⓒ Ⓓ	24	Ⓐ Ⓑ Ⓒ Ⓓ
5	Ⓐ Ⓑ Ⓒ Ⓓ	15	Ⓐ Ⓑ Ⓒ Ⓓ	25	Ⓐ Ⓑ Ⓒ Ⓓ
6	Ⓐ Ⓑ Ⓒ Ⓓ	16	Ⓐ Ⓑ Ⓒ Ⓓ	26	Ⓐ Ⓑ Ⓒ Ⓓ
7	Ⓐ Ⓑ Ⓒ Ⓓ	17	Ⓐ Ⓑ Ⓒ Ⓓ	27	Ⓐ Ⓑ Ⓒ Ⓓ
8	Ⓐ Ⓑ Ⓒ Ⓓ	18	Ⓐ Ⓑ Ⓒ Ⓓ	28	Ⓐ Ⓑ Ⓒ Ⓓ
9	Ⓐ Ⓑ Ⓒ Ⓓ	19	Ⓐ Ⓑ Ⓒ Ⓓ		
10	Ⓐ Ⓑ Ⓒ Ⓓ	20	Ⓐ Ⓑ Ⓒ Ⓓ		

Part I. Reading

53 questions (47 scored), 64 minutes

Text Messaging

To send a text message to a landline number, open your device in landscape mode and press TXT. Enter the landline number and press OK. Type the message and press OK again. You will receive an Opt-In message. Press V to view the message, and then press R to reply.

To send a text message to a wireless device, open your device in landscape mode and press TXT. Enter the phone number or e-mail address of the recipient in the To: field using the QWERTY keyboard. If you have contacts stored in your Contact list, you will see a list of partially matched names in the drop-down box. Use the directional arrows to select a contact. Press OK. Enter your message in the TXT field, and press OK to send.

The next five questions are based on this passage.

1. The reader can infer that this passage was taken from which of the following?

   A) A comic book
   B) A manual
   C) An editorial
   D) A textbook

2. The passage is reflective of which of the following types of text structure?

   A) Cause-effect
   B) Sequence
   C) Definition and examples
   D) Reasons and examples

3. Which of the following is the intention of the passage?

   A) To persuade
   B) To entertain
   C) To reflect
   D) To instruct

4. Which of the following inferences may logically be drawn from the passage?

   A) Most recipients of text messages have landlines.
   B) Text messages cannot be sent to landlines.
   C) Text messages may be sent in more than one way.
   D) The device may only be opened in landscape mode.

GO ON TO THE NEXT PAGE

5. The passage is reflective of which of the following types of writing?

   A) Narrative
   B) Descriptive
   C) Technical
   D) Persuasive

The Visitor

We had lived in the little house for two years before we started noticing signs that we were sharing the yard with something large. First, the garbage cans were knocked around.

"It's a raccoon," said Pete sagely.

Next, we woke to find that the iron poles that secured the birdfeeders to the ground were bent in half. The seeds were gone, and there were claw marks on the wooden feeders.

"Well, maybe it's not a raccoon," Pete admitted.

When the snow started that year, our guesses were confirmed. I pointed to the large prints that led from the closed garage door back up into the woods behind the house.

"That's some bear!" Pete whistled.

That night, he came home with a box. Unloading it on the dining room table, he pieced together a couple of odd-looking cameras.

"They're trail cams. Infrared," he explained. I followed him outside as he hung the cameras on two nearby trees.

The next morning, the trail cam offered confirmation. In a series of shots, we could see the bear in silhouette as he (or she) wandered down the hill, scratched at the garage door once or twice, climbed the stairs to the back deck, sat there for a while rocking back and forth, and ambled slowly back into the woods.

Pete explained that feeding the bear amounted to baiting him and was frowned on by the authorities. "As it gets colder," he said, "the bear will hibernate, and we can put the birdfeeders back up. Right now, we're better off keeping all food out of his way." Sharing our space with the natural world is always a challenge.

The next seven questions are based on this passage.

   6. Which detail in the third paragraph *most clearly* leads Pete to conclude that the visitor is not a raccoon?

   A) Claw marks
   B) Wooden feeders
   C) Seeds gone
   D) Bent poles

GO ON TO THE NEXT PAGE

7. Which of the following sentences states an opinion?

A) First, the garbage cans were knocked around.
B) The seeds were gone, and there were claw marks on the wooden feeders.
C) I followed him outside as he hung the cameras on two nearby trees.
D) "Right now, we're better off keeping all food out of his way."

8. The passage is reflective of which of the following types of writing?

A) Narrative
B) Expository
C) Technical
D) Persuasive

9. Which of the following is an example of a summary sentence in the passage?

A) The next morning, the trail cam offered confirmation.
B) "Well, maybe it's not a raccoon," Pete admitted.
C) When the snow started that year, our guesses were confirmed.
D) Sharing our space with the natural world is always a challenge.

10. Based on the final paragraph, how do the writer and Pete feel toward the bear?

A) Nervous
B) Fearful
C) Accepting
D) Annoyed

11. Which of the following describes the word *nature* as it relates to the passage?

A) Theme
B) Topic
C) Main idea
D) Supporting detail

12. What does the author intend to do with the three short paragraphs (second, fourth, and sixth) that contain Pete's statements about the visitor?

A) Persuade
B) Inform
C) Entertain
D) Reflect

GO ON TO THE NEXT PAGE

As you use your circular saw, stand to the side, in case the wood kicks back. Start the blade before it connects to the wood. Guide the saw, don't push it. The blade will continue to spin after you release it, so be careful.

The next two questions are based on this passage.

13. Based on the passage, which of the following is a logical prediction of what the author will tell the reader to do next?

    A) Put on some protective gloves and goggles.
    B) Carefully check the sharpness of the blade.
    C) Let the blade stop before removing it from the wood.
    D) Avoid knots and burls in the wood that you cut.

14. Based on a prior knowledge of literature, the reader can infer that this passage was taken from which of the following?

    A) A letter to the editor
    B) A work of fiction
    C) A children's magazine
    D) A how-to manual

15. A student studying for a test from a textbook wonders which chapters are most pertinent to the test's subject matter. Where should the student look to find out?

    A) In the index
    B) In the table of contents
    C) In the preface
    D) In the glossary

16. Read and follow the directions below.

    1. Andy, Bret, Carrie, and Dave are standing in line in that order, with Andy first in line.

    2. Carrie steps behind Dave.

    3. Dave steps in front of Bret.

    4. Andy steps behind Carrie.

    What is the order of the four people now?

    A) Andy, Carrie, Dave, Bret
    B) Bret, Carrie, Andy, Dave
    C) Dave, Bret, Carrie, Andy
    D) Carrie, Andy, Dave, Bret

GO ON TO THE NEXT PAGE

17. **Administrative support specialist:** Begin with the basics of keyboarding, letter writing, business English, filing, and the use of office machines including calculators, photocopiers, telephones, and fax machines. This training program will focus on the skills necessary for mid- to upper-level support positions such as Administrative Assistant, Executive Secretary, Legal Secretary, and Medical Secretary. We will focus on Word proficiency as well as training in Excel, PowerPoint, and Access. M–F 8:30–3:30, 24 weeks. Tuition: $6,400.

Who would most benefit from this course?

A) A nurse wishing to train on PowerPoint and Access
B) A low-level office worker hoping to advance
C) A secretary well versed in Word and Excel
D) A student working on a degree in hospital administration

18. Obviously she doesn't know the answer; her <u>nebulous</u> reply left us completely in the dark.

Which of the following is the definition of the word *nebulous*?

A) Compelling
B) Unfounded
C) Agile
D) Vague

GO ON TO THE NEXT PAGE

KITCHEN DESIGN & REMODELING

CK Construction 2 Divan St 555-3910

Foster Custom Kitchens

    24 State St 555-6789

Willet Kitchen & Bath 129 Bly Pl . . . 555-6822

KITCHEN EQUIPMENT

Cookout Landreau Mall 555-2566

Miko Bar & Kitchen 32 State St 555-1700

Sanduhra Foods 421 Burr St 555-0909

KUNG FU INSTRUCTION

See Martial Arts Instruction

LABORATORIES—CLINICAL

Asthma & Allergy Assoc. Durham Pl . . . 555-2770

Kiowa Medical Center State St. . . 555-4300

Landreau Mall 555-4311

> **FOSTER CUSTOM KITCHENS**
> The finest in cabinetry for over
> 50 years!

> **LABORATORIES—DENTAL**
> Asok Dental 495 Marco Blvd . . . 555-2780
> Canto Family Dentistry
>   422 Burr St 555-8998
> Small Dental Lab 877 Fortuna St . . 555-0065
> **LABORATORIES—TESTING**
> Enviro Control 8712 Rte 14 555-8909
> Kiowa Medical Center State St . . . 555-4300
> Microvac 225 University Pl 555-1330

> **CANTO FAMILY DENTISTRY**
> On-site lab for same-day service!
> Full-service dentistry for the whole
> family 555-8998

The next two questions are based on this sample yellow page.

19. A customer wishes to test the level of radon in her basement. Which number would she most logically call?

    A) 555-8909
    B) 555-4300
    C) 555-0065
    D) 555-2770

20. Which facility has a branch office at the local mall?

    A) Asok Dental
    B) Asthma & Allergy Associates
    C) Kiowa Medical Center
    D) Canto Family Dentistry

21.

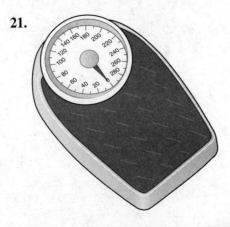

GO ON TO THE NEXT PAGE

What is the maximum weight the scale on the previous page will measure?

A) Just over 130 pounds
B) Just over 250 pounds
C) Just over 280 pounds
D) Just over 320 pounds

22.

Nutrition Facts

Serving size 3 oz (85 g)
Servings per container 1

Amount per serving

Calories 180	Calories from fat 90
	% Daily value*

Total fat 10 g	15%
Saturated fat 40 g	20%
Trans fat 0.5 g	
Cholesterol 70 mg	23%
Sodium 60 mg	3%
Total carbohydrate 0 g	0%
Dietary fiber 0 g	0%
Sugars 0 g	
Protein 22 g	

Vitamin A 0%	•	Vitamin C 0%
Calcium 2%	•	Iron 15%

• Percent daily values are based on a 2,000 calorie diet. Your daily values may be higher or lower depending on your calorie needs:

	Calories:	2,000	2,500
Total fat	Less than	65 g	80 g
Saturated fat	Less than	20 g	25 g
Cholesterol	Less than	300 mg	300 mg
Sodium	Less than	2,400 mg	2,400 mg
Total carbohydrate		300 g	375 g
Dietary fiber		25 g	30 g

Calories per gram:
  Fat 9 • Carbohydrate 4 • Protein 4

A customer eating one of these snacks should probably limit which type of intake for the rest of the day?

A) Sodium
B) Calcium
C) Cholesterol
D) Vitamin C

GO ON TO THE NEXT PAGE

Directions: Apply the gel on the gingival <u>margin</u> around the selected teeth using the blunt-tipped applicator included in the package. Wait 30 seconds; then fill the periodontal pockets with the gel using the blunt-tipped applicator until the gel becomes visible at the gingival margin. Wait another 30 seconds before starting treatment. A longer waiting time does not enhance the anesthesia. Anesthetic effect, as assessed by probing of pocket depths, lasts approximately 20 minutes (individual overall range 14–31 minutes). If the anesthesia starts to wear off, the gel may be reapplied if needed.

The next two questions are based on this passage.

23. Which of the following is the definition of the word *margin*?

    A) Edge
    B) Grease
    C) Incisor
    D) Cavity

24. If you wait 70 seconds instead of 60 seconds to begin treatment, what will happen?

    A) The anesthetic will take stronger effect.
    B) The anesthetic will wear off entirely.
    C) You will waste 10 seconds of the drug's duration.
    D) You will be unable to administer a second dose.

Do you fall asleep often during the day? After eating, do you feel suddenly drowsy? Does laughing too hard cause you momentarily to lose the ability to move? Does anyone else in your family share these symptoms? You may suffer from narcolepsy. This chronic, incurable condition is apparently caused by reduced amounts of the brain protein called hypocretin.

The next two questions are based on this passage.

25. What is the author's apparent purpose for writing this paragraph about narcolepsy?

    A) To explain cause and effect
    B) To give step-by-step instructions
    C) To reflect on a personal problem
    D) To present an opinion

26. In the context of the passage, does the mention of laughing too hard constitute a topic, a main idea, a theme, or supporting details?

    A) Topic
    B) Main idea
    C) Theme
    D) Supporting details

GO ON TO THE NEXT PAGE

27. A person about to transfer jobs would like to hold a moving sale and hopes to alert potential buyers. Which department of the newspaper should he contact?

  A) Editorial
  B) Business
  C) Local news
  D) Classified

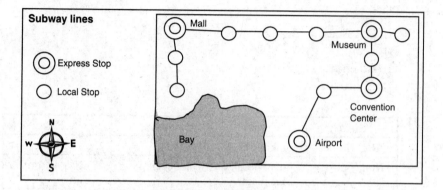

The next two questions are based on this map.

28. Stella and Della set out from the mall to the airport. Stella takes the local line, and Della takes the express line. How many more stops does Stella have than Della?

  A) Eight more
  B) Seven more
  C) Six more
  D) Five more

29. A man starts at a local stop and heads north one stop to an express stop. He then takes the express train one stop west. Where does he leave the train?

  A) At the museum
  B) At the mall
  C) At the airport
  D) At the convention center

GO ON TO THE NEXT PAGE

30. Chapter 5: The Olympian Gods

    A. Odysseus
    B. Zeus
    C. Athena
    D. Aphrodite

Analyze the headings above. Which of the following headings is out of place?

A) Odysseus
B) Zeus
C) Athena
D) Aphrodite

31.

Store	Colors	Size	Price
ABC Home	pink floral	twin, king	$69.99–$79.99
Homebody	green floral, blue plaid	twin, queen, king	$129.99–$149.99
Excelsior	white stripe, yellow floral	double, queen	$89.50–$95.50
The Bedroom	red stripe, gray stripe, blue stripe	queen, king	$99.99–$109.99

A customer wants a queen-sized comforter in a floral pattern for under $100. Which store's product suits her needs?

A) ABC Home
B) Homebody
C) Excelsior
D) The Bedroom

32. A traveler planning a world tour wonders whether it is more reasonable to travel from east to west or from west to east. Which resource might help the traveler make a decision?

A) A road map
B) A world atlas
C) A travel brochure
D) An encyclopedia

33. Appetite control, 187
Appetite suppressants, 181
Arteriosclerosis, 250
Arthritis, 280
Artificial insemination, 310–312

GO ON TO THE NEXT PAGE

In the book whose index is excerpted on the previous page, which pages probably contain the chapter on diet and nutrition?

A) 165–190
B) 191–224
C) 225–258
D) 259–290

34. Starting image

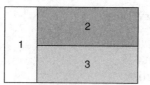

Start with the shape pictured above. Follow the directions to alter its appearance.

1. Move section 1 from the left edge of the shape to the right.
2. Rotate the entire shape 90 degrees to the left.

Which of the following represents the shape after these alterations?

A)

B)

C)

D)

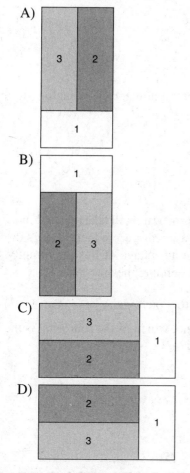

GO ON TO THE NEXT PAGE

35. The banquet was _____, with foods from dozens of caterers.

Which word could complete the sentence above with the most positive connotation?

A) excessive
B) lavish
C) wasteful
D) overindulgent

36. Chapter 8: Fairy Tales

    1. European Tales
        A. Norse
        B. English
        C. French
        D. _____
        E. German

Examine the headings above. Based on what you see, which of the following is a reasonable heading to insert in the blank spot?

A) Japanese
B) Native American
C) African
D) Portuguese

The following memo was sent by the director of technology to office managers.

To: Managerial Staff

From: Paul Litvak

Re: Training

Training on the new information system software will take place Monday and Wednesday from noon until 3. We are paying for <u>accredited</u> trainers to come down from Minneapolis, so please take advantage of this opportunity. You may sign up for one or both sessions by sending me an e-mail.

The next two questions are based on this passage.

37. Based on the context of this memo, which of the following is the best definition of the underlined word?

A) Qualified
B) Praiseworthy
C) Faithful
D) Underwritten

GO ON TO THE NEXT PAGE

38. What does the author think about the training?

    A) It is overpriced.
    B) It is not difficult.
    C) It is worth taking.
    D) It is insignificant.

from Women and Economics

by Charlotte Perkins Gilman

Recognizing her intense feeling on moral lines, and seeing in her the rigidly preserved virtues of faith, submission, and self-sacrifice—qualities which in the dark ages were held to be the first of virtues,—we have agreed of late years to call woman the moral superior of man. But the ceaseless growth of human life, social life, has developed in him new virtues, later, higher, more needful; and the moral nature of woman, as maintained in this rudimentary stage by her economic dependence, is a continual check to the progress of the human soul. The main feature of her life—the restriction of her range and duty to the love and service of her own immediate family—acts upon us continually as a retarding influence, hindering the expansion of the spirit of social love and service on which our very lives depend. It keeps the moral standard of the patriarchal era still before us, and blinds our eyes to the full duty of man.

The next two questions are based on this passage.

39. Which best identifies the theme of this passage?

    A) Faith and self-sacrifice
    B) Justice and goodness
    C) The road to financial self-reliance
    D) Dependence as a moral impediment

40. Which of the following details from the passage best indicates its historical context?

    A) The mention of the Dark Ages
    B) The emphasis on morality
    C) The focus on restriction of women
    D) The interest in social life

GO ON TO THE NEXT PAGE

41. Read and follow the directions below.

1. Imagine a train running east and west among four towns spaced five miles apart.
2. The train starts at Addison and travels west to Barnard.
3. It continues west 5 miles to Compton.
4. It continues west 5 miles to Daly and turns around.
5. The train continues back and forth for another 30 miles.

At which town does the train finally stop?

A) Addison
B) Barnard
C) Compton
D) Daly

42. A nurse uses a search engine to locate information on the causes of rosacea. Which of the following websites is most likely to be helpful?

A) www.rosacea.org/patients/materials/understanding/causes.php
B) www.webmd.com/skin-problems-and.../rosacea-symptoms
C) www.managemyrosacea.com
D) www.rosaceatopicaltreatment.com

43.

On the thermometer above, what is the current temperature in degrees Fahrenheit?

GO ON TO THE NEXT PAGE

A) 24°
B) 28°
C) 76°
D) 80°

Store	Price per 20-Pound Bag	Shipping and Handling
Pets and More	$25	50¢ per pound
Feathered Friends	$30	Free
Birdland	$22	$5 for first 5 pounds, free after that
Feather Your Nest	$26	25¢ per pound

The next two questions are based on this pricing chart.

44. Which store offers the best deal on purchasing and shipping a 20-pound bag of seed?

   A) Pets and More
   B) Feathered Friends
   C) Birdland
   D) Feather Your Nest

45. Jason has $100 to spend, not counting tax. If he drives to the store rather than having the seed shipped, which stores will allow him to buy at least four bags of seed?

   A) Pets and More and Birdland
   B) Feathered Friends and Feather Your Nest
   C) Pets and More and Feathered Friends
   D) All except Feathered Friends

GO ON TO THE NEXT PAGE

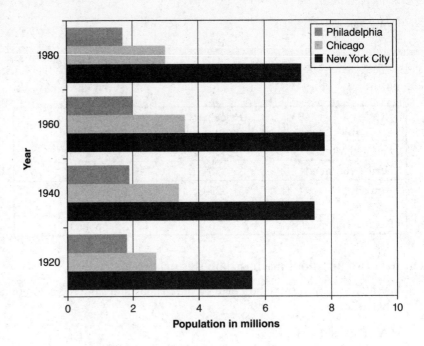

Population in millions

The next two questions are based on this graph.

46. About how much greater was the population of New York than that of Philadelphia in 1960?

A) A little under 4 million
B) A little under 5 million
C) A little under 6 million
D) A little under 7 million

47. In which year did Chicago have the greatest population?

A) 1920
B) 1940
C) 1960
D) 1980

48. Having completed their dance, the tom turkeys <u>repair</u> to the back field to wait for the hens' response.

Based on the context of the sentence above, which of the following is the definition of the underlined word?

A) Fix up
B) Amend
C) Renovate
D) Set off

GO ON TO THE NEXT PAGE

Eco-Friendly Weed Killers

Vinegar is an effective and risk-free weed killer. Its application in moderation kills weeds without harming anything else. Adding a little salt to the vinegar can ensure that the weed killing is permanent. Just add one cup of salt to a gallon of vinegar, stir in a tablespoon of liquid dishwashing detergent, and use in a spray bottle on those difficult weeds.

If you coat the weeds with this mixture on a sunny day, the plants will die in a matter of days and will not return. Be sure to label your mixture clearly and store it out of reach in a garage or basement.

The next two questions are based on this passage.

49. Which of the following statements would most contradict the writer's argument?

 A) Without the addition of salt, vinegar is not a permanent solution for weeds.
 B) Liquid detergent can help the vinegar and salt stick to leaves and stems.
 C) Plants may grow up between patio stones and cause them to shift.
 D) The solution kills all plants it touches, not just the weeds you want eliminated.

50. Which of the following conclusions is best supported by the passage?

 A) Weeds may return no matter what you do to get rid of them.
 B) It is possible to eliminate weeds without using toxic chemicals.
 C) Difficult weeds are a challenge for any gardener or homeowner.
 D) It is not possible to get rid of weeds on a humid or rainy day.

51. Doris had not yet received her degree; _____, her advisor encouraged her to apply to the prestigious graduate program.

 Which word or phrase would best complete the sentence?

 A) nevertheless
 B) accordingly
 C) consequently
 D) for that reason

GO ON TO THE NEXT PAGE

52. Which of these statements about rubella is a fact?

A) Rubella is not as dangerous as rubeola (measles).
B) Pregnant women should protect themselves from rubella.
C) Rubella is the number one cause of congenital deafness.
D) The infection is mild but may have some nasty complications.

53. The bin marked *hazardous waste* contains corrosive and reactive chemicals and materials.

How are italics used in the sentence?

A) To stress important words
B) To signify words in another language
C) To identify the title of a work
D) To delineate a word used as a label

STOP. THIS IS THE END OF PART I.

Part II. Mathematics

36 items (32 scored), 54 minutes

1. Express $\dfrac{9}{25}$ as a decimal.

   A) 0.09
   B) 0.18
   C) 0.9
   D) 0.36

2. Farmer Brown has four wooden posts that average 5 feet tall. If he cut 6 inches off each of three posts to have the 52-inch fence post height he wanted, how much must he cut off the fourth post to have a fourth 52-inch post?

   A) 6 inches
   B) 10 inches
   C) 14 inches
   D) 18 inches

3. At the book sale, Geoff paid 35 cents apiece for five paperbacks and $2.50 apiece for three hardcover books. He gave the clerk a $10 bill. How much change did he receive?

   A) $0.50
   B) $0.75
   C) $1.25
   D) $1.75

4. What is the product of the numbers 0.05×0.22?

   A) 1.1
   B) 0.11
   C) 0.011
   D) 0.0011

5. How many kilograms are there in 11 pounds? (Note: 1 kilogram = 2.2 pounds.)

   A) 5 kilograms
   B) 5.5 kilograms
   C) 22.2 kilograms
   D) 24.2 kilograms

GO ON TO THE NEXT PAGE

6. The Soap Factory is selling three bars of almond-scented soaps for $2.58. What would it cost to buy five bars of soap?

A) $3.30
B) $3.80
C) $4.30
D) $4.80

7. Of the 1,525 homes sold by Homestyle Realty last year, Clara sold 244. What percentage of the homes did she sell?

A) 16%
B) 18%
C) 22%
D) 24%

8. $(2x + 2)(2x - 2)$

Simplify the expression above. Which of the following is correct?

A) $4x^2 - 4x - 4$
B) $4x^2 - 2x - 4$
C) $4x^2 + 4x - 4$
D) $4x^2 - 4$

9. What is the perimeter of a rectangular field that is 25 yards wide and 40 yards long?

A) 65 yards
B) 90 yards
C) 130 yards
D) 1,000 yards

GO ON TO THE NEXT PAGE

10.

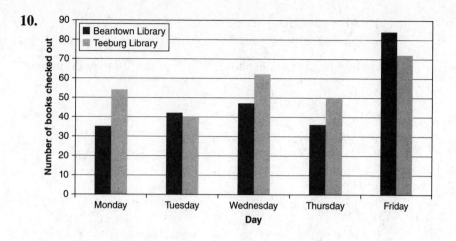

The graph above shows the numbers of books checked out at two libraries over the course of five days.

On Friday, the difference between the numbers of books checked out at the two libraries was

A) less than 10.
B) between 10 and 15.
C) between 15 and 20.
D) greater than 20.

11.

Year	Price per Gallon
1950	26.4¢
1970	37¢
1980	108¢

This table shows the cost of gasoline in three different eras.

In 1950, what was the greatest number of gallons of gas you could buy for $5?

A) 12 gallons
B) 18 gallons
C) 24 gallons
D) 30 gallons

GO ON TO THE NEXT PAGE

12. $4\dfrac{1}{8} \div \dfrac{1}{4}$

Simplify the expression above. Which of the following is correct?

A) $\dfrac{11}{32}$

B) $4\dfrac{1}{2}$

C) $16\dfrac{1}{2}$

D) 264

13. Luisa bought books for her classes at costs of $50.55, $35.00, $65.00, $75.50, and $22.50. What was the median cost of her books?

A) $49.71
B) $50.55
C) $53.00
D) $65.00

14. Which answer is correct for the product of 0.6×0.06?

A) 0.0036
B) 0.036
C) 0.36
D) 3.6

15. How many grams are there in 14 kilograms?

A) 1.4 grams
B) 140 grams
C) 1,400 grams
D) 14,000 grams

GO ON TO THE NEXT PAGE

16.

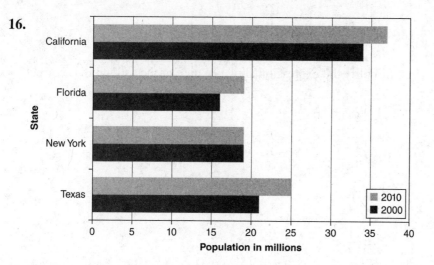

The graph above shows the populations of the most populous U.S. states in 2000 and 2010.

If displayed trends continue, which would you expect to happen by 2020?

A) Texas will surpass California in population.
B) Florida will surpass New York in population.
C) Texas's population will decline, and California's will increase.
D) California's population will decline, and Texas's will increase.

17.

Day	Wind Speed in kph
Monday	28
Tuesday	26
Wednesday	20
Thursday	14
Friday	42

This table shows the wind speed in kilometers per hour at Buzzville Airport.

One knot = 1.852 kph. If the crosswind limit for aircraft at Buzzville Airport is about 25 knots, on which days could aircraft *not* land at the airport?

A) Friday only
B) Monday and Friday
C) Monday, Tuesday, and Friday
D) Aircraft could land on all five days.

GO ON TO THE NEXT PAGE

18. $5\dfrac{2}{3} + \dfrac{6}{7}$

Simplify the expression above. Which of the following is correct?

A) $6\dfrac{1}{21}$

B) $6\dfrac{1}{7}$

C) $6\dfrac{3}{14}$

D) $6\dfrac{11}{21}$

19. $(2 \times 3) + 6 + (5 \times 6) - 2$

Simplify the expression above. Which of the following is correct?

A) 100
B) 50
C) 46
D) 40

20. As time passes, eggs begin to hatch.

Which is the dependent variable in the statement above?

A) Hatching of eggs
B) Number of eggs
C) Time
D) Temperature

21. Which of the following decimal numbers is approximately equal to $\sqrt{63}$?

A) 7.15
B) 7.75
C) 7.95
D) 8.05

22. Nurse Lamont ordered 12 cartons of pipettes for the lab at a cost of $24.95 per carton. Which of the following is an accurate estimate of the cost of the pipettes?

A) $250
B) $300
C) $350
D) $400

GO ON TO THE NEXT PAGE

23. $4\dfrac{5}{6} \times 1\dfrac{1}{8}$

Simplify the expression above. Which of the following is correct?

A) $5\dfrac{7}{16}$

B) $5\dfrac{11}{24}$

C) $5\dfrac{1}{4}$

D) $4\dfrac{5}{48}$

24.

Deposits	Withdrawals	Beginning Balance
		$1,280.75
$989.25		
	$20.00	
	$50.00	
	$675.00	
$989.25		
	$50.00	
	$25.30	

This table shows Al's checking account during the month of December.

What was the balance in Al's account at the end of December?

A) $1,158.20
B) $1,449.70
C) $2,438.95
D) $3,259.25

25. What is the product of 5.2×2.5?

A) 0.013
B) 0.13
C) 1.3
D) 13

GO ON TO THE NEXT PAGE

26. The weights of newborns born at Loving Care Hospital Friday averaged 3.2 kg. If the newborns weighed 2.8 kg, 3.8 kg, 2.9 kg, 3.1 kg, and x, what was the value of x?

A) 3.1 kg
B) 3.2 kg
C) 3.3 kg
D) 3.4 kg

27. What number is 125% of 75?

A) 56.25
B) 78.5
C) 93.75
D) 98.5

28. In a scale drawing for a garden, 2 cm = 1 m. If the garden measures 8 cm by 10 cm in the drawing, how large will it be in reality?

A) 2 m by 3 m
B) 4 m by 5 m
C) 8 m by 10 m
D) 16 m by 20 m

29. A nurse is measuring cough medicine for a patient's treatment. Which would be the most accurate tool to use for this task?

A) Beaker
B) Measuring cup
C) Measuring spoon
D) Graduated cylinder

30. $|-2| \times |3|$

Simplify the expression above.

A) 6
B) −6
C) 1
D) −1

31. John's height in inches, h, is twice that of his nephew's, c, minus 20 inches.

Which of the following algebraic expressions best represents the statement above?

A) $c = 2(h - 20)$
B) $h = 2c - 20$
C) $h - 20 = c$
D) $h = 2 \times 20c$

GO ON TO THE NEXT PAGE

32. Order this list of numbers from least to greatest.

$-17, \dfrac{34}{2}, -17.5, 16.9$

   A) $-17, -17.5, \dfrac{34}{2}, 16.9$

   B) $-17.5, -17, \dfrac{34}{2}, 16.9$

   C) $-17, -17.5, 16.9, \dfrac{34}{2}$

   D) $-17.5, -17, 16.9, \dfrac{34}{2}$

33. Which type of graph would best indicate the percentage of a college class entering various careers?

   A) Line graph
   B) Histogram
   C) Circle graph
   D) Scatter plot

34. A touchdown plus kick is good for 7 points. A field goal is good for 3 points. If Jonny's team is down by 17 points, which combination of touchdowns and field goals provides the minimum points needed to win the game, assuming that the other team does not score?

   A) 1 touchdown and 3 field goals
   B) 2 touchdowns and 1 field goal
   C) 2 touchdowns and 2 field goals
   D) 3 touchdowns

GO ON TO THE NEXT PAGE

35.

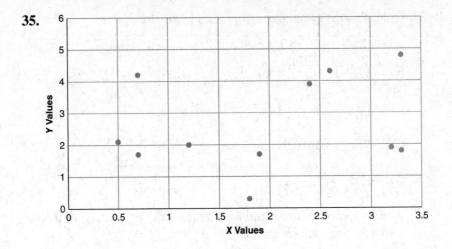

What can you conclude about the relationship between *x* and *y* on the graph above?

A) As *x* increases, *y* decreases.
B) As *x* decreases, *y* increases.
C) As *x* increases, *y* increases.
D) No relationship exists.

36. At the fair, ice cream cones are $2, and sprinkles are 50 cents. A father buys his children and their friends several cones, some with sprinkles.

Which of the following algebraic expressions represents what he pays?

A) $x + y$
B) $2x + 2.5y$
C) $2x + y/2$
D) $2x + 50y$

> ### STOP. THIS IS THE END OF PART II.

Part III. Science

53 items (47 scored), 63 minutes

1. The skull is _____ to the brain.

   Which of the following correctly completes the sentence above?

   A) medial
   B) superficial
   C) inferior
   D) intermediate

2. How does a sagittal section divide the body?

   A) Into right and left regions
   B) Into upper and lower regions
   C) Into front and back regions
   D) Between the dorsal and ventral cavities

3. While conducting an experiment, a scientist makes inferences from data to recommend a revised experimental focus. This action corresponds to which of the following steps in the scientific method?

   A) Formulating a hypothesis
   B) Collecting data
   C) Analyzing data
   D) Drawing a conclusion

4. The esophagus is part of the _____ system.

   Which of the following correctly completes the sentence above?

   A) endocrine
   B) digestive
   C) respiratory
   D) nervous

GO ON TO THE NEXT PAGE

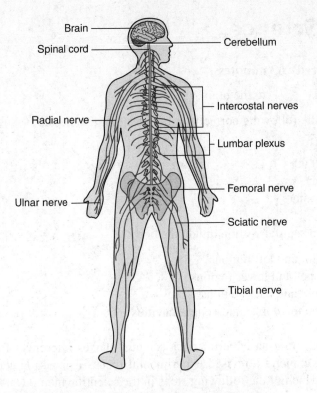

Brain
Cerebellum
Spinal cord
Intercostal nerves
Radial nerve
Lumbar plexus
Femoral nerve
Ulnar nerve
Sciatic nerve
Tibial nerve

The next two questions are based on this diagram.

5. The part of the nervous system shown in this diagram is primarily

    A) somatic.
    B) autonomic.
    C) sympathetic.
    D) parasympathetic.

6. Where would a herniated lumbar disc most likely create pain?

    A) Along the radial nerve
    B) Within the spinal cord
    C) Along the sciatic nerve
    D) Along the tibial nerve

7. Empirical data is derived from _____ and _____.

Which of the following correctly completes the sentence above?

    A) observation; experimentation
    B) postulating; theorizing
    C) common sense; repetition
    D) conceptualizing; modeling

GO ON TO THE NEXT PAGE

8.

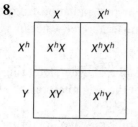

	X	X^h
X^h	X^hX	X^hX^h
Y	XY	X^hY

Hemophilia is a sex-linked trait. In the example above of a male with hemophilia and a female carrier, what ratio of the offspring would be predicted to neither carry nor manifest the disease?

A) 0 female : 1 male
B) 1 female : 1 male
C) 1 female : 0 male
D) 2 females : 1 male

9.

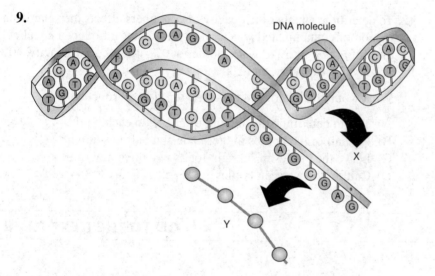

DNA molecule

In the diagram above, what product is represented by Y?

A) Ribosome
B) mRNA
C) Uracil
D) Protein

10. In a graph showing the growth of bacterial colonies, what might be another term for "Log phase"?

A) Decline phase
B) Exponential growth
C) Stationary phase
D) Maximum phase

GO ON TO THE NEXT PAGE

11. How should a researcher test the hypothesis that radiation from cell phones is significant enough to raise the temperature of water in a test tube?

A) Dial a cell phone that rests beside a test tube of water, let it ring for 2 minutes, and record the temperature of the water before and after the 2-minute interval.

B) Dial a cell phone that rests beside a test tube of water, let it ring for 2, 3, and 4 minutes, and record the temperature of the water before and after each interval.

C) Use three different brands of cell phone; dial each as it rests beside its own test tube of water, let it ring for 2 minutes, and record the temperature of the water before and after the 2-minute interval.

D) Use three different brands of cell phone, dial each and let one ring for 2 minutes, one for 3 minutes, and one for 4 minutes; record the temperature of the water before and after each interval.

12. To determine whether the opacity of containers affects the solar disinfection of contaminated water, an experimenter introduced equal cultures of *E. coli* into 1-L water bottles at 0% opacity, 25% opacity, 50% opacity, 75% opacity, and 100% opacity.

What would be the logical next step for the experimenter?

A) Test to determine the amount of *E. coli* in each bottle.
B) Put half of the bottles in the shade and half in sunlight.
C) Leave the bottles in sunlight for an equal amount of time.
D) Culture the water in bottles at 0%, 50%, and 100% opacity.

GO ON TO THE NEXT PAGE

13.

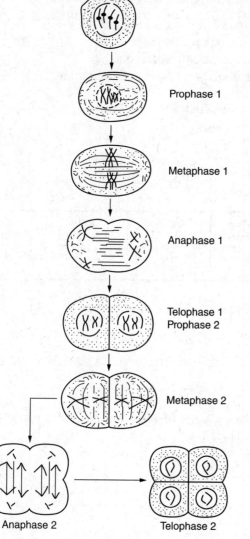

What does this diagram show?

A) Catabolic reaction
B) Anabolic reaction
C) Meiosis
D) Mitosis

14. Beriberi is a disease caused by lack of

A) vitamin C.
B) niacin.
C) thiamine.
D) protein.

GO ON TO THE NEXT PAGE

15. Why are diuretics ineffective as a weight-loss product?

A) Side effects include increased calorie intake.
B) The drugs may not be used by older adults.
C) Diuretics do not increase the metabolic rate.
D) The weight loss is temporary and unrelated to fat.

16. Which one has the highest density?

A) Mist
B) Water
C) Steam
D) Ice

17.

Gas	Carbon monoxide	Carbon dioxide	Sulfur dioxide	Methane
Molar Mass	28.00 g/mol	44.01 g/mol	64.07 g/mol	16.042 g/mol

Which would you expect to diffuse most rapidly?

A) Carbon monoxide
B) Carbon dioxide
C) Sulfur dioxide
D) Methane

18. Which of the following parts of the brain has the most to do with coordination and balance?

A) Parietal lobe
B) Cerebellum
C) Amygdala
D) Temporal lobe

19. Which would be a normal amount of urine produced daily by a healthy adult?

A) 100 mL
B) 300 mL
C) 1 L
D) 3 L

20. Where do lymphocytes go to mature into T cells?

A) Thalamus
B) Thymus
C) Thyroid
D) Testes

GO ON TO THE NEXT PAGE

21.

PERIODIC TABLE OF THE ELEMENTS

1 H																	2 He
3 Li	4 Be											5 B	6 C	7 N	8 O	9 F	10 Ne
11 Na	12 Mg											13 Al	14 Si	15 P	16 S	17 Ci	18 Ar
19 K	20 Ca	21 Sc	22 Ti	23 V	24 Cr	25 Mn	26 Fe	27 Co	28 Ni	29 Cu	30 Zn	31 Ga	32 Ge	33 As	34 Se	35 Br	36 Kr
37 Rb	38 Sr	39 Y	40 Z	41 Nb	42 Mo	43 Tc	44 Ru	45 Rh	46 Pd	47 Ag	48 Cd	49 In	50 Sn	51 Sb	52 Te	53 I	54 Xe
55 Cs	56 Ba	see below	72 Hf	73 Ta	74 W	75 Re	76 Os	77 It	78 Pt	79 Au	80 Hg	81 Ti	82 Pb	83 Bi	84 Po	85 At	86 Rn
87 Fr	88 Ra	see below	104 Rf	105 Db	106 Sg	107 Bh	108 Hs	109 Mt	110 Ds	111 Rg	112 Uub	113 Uut	114 Uuq	115 Uup	116 Uuh	117 Uus	118 Uuo

■ = Alkali Metals   ▨ = Halogens   ▨ = Noble Gases

RARE EARTH ELEMENTS

Lanthanides	57 La	58 Ce	59 Pr	60 Nd	61 Pm	62 Sm	63 Eu	64 Gd	65 Tb	66 Dy	67 Ho	68 Er	69 Tm	70 Yb	71 Lu
Actinides	89 Ac	90 Th	91 Pa	92 U	93 Np	94 Pu	95 Am	96 Cm	97 Bk	98 Cf	99 Es	100 Fm	101 Md	102 No	103 Lr

Which gives the number of protons in the atomic nucleus of an alkali metal?

A) 9
B) 10
C) 11
D) 12

GO ON TO THE NEXT PAGE

22.

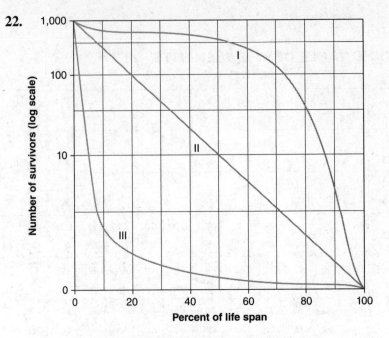

Survivorship curve I would be most applicable to

A) a species with few offspring that receive good care.
B) a species with a fairly constant death rate.
C) a species with many offspring that receive little care.
D) There is no way to determine this.

GO ON TO THE NEXT PAGE

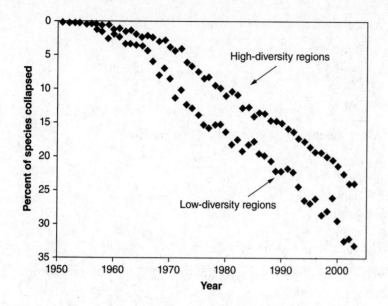

The next two questions are based on this graph.

23. According to this graph, which statement is true?

   A) Loss of species is faster in high-diversity regions.
   B) Loss of species is faster in low-diversity regions.
   C) Loss of species does not correlate with diversity.
   D) Loss of species is caused by increased diversity.

24. In the graph above, the correlation between species collapse and time is

   A) direct.
   B) scattered.
   C) inverse.
   D) nonexistent.

25. How would you describe the connective tissue found in tendons?

   A) Loose regular
   B) Dense regular
   C) Loose irregular
   D) Dense irregular

26. When an acid and a base neutralize each other, which products are formed?

   A) A metal and water
   B) A nonmetal and water
   C) A salt and water
   D) An ion and water

GO ON TO THE NEXT PAGE

27. Where is the epidermis thickest?

A) Buttocks
B) Scalp
C) Cheek
D) Palm

28. Where are the sweat glands most concentrated?

A) Feet
B) Face
C) Back
D) Armpit

29. The spleen is located to the _____ of the stomach.

Which of the following correctly completes the sentence above?

A) rear
B) front
C) left
D) right

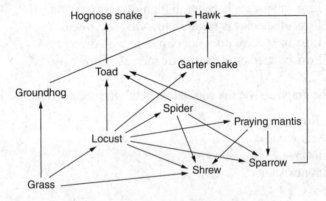

The next two questions are based on this diagram.

30. A disease causing die-out at the second trophic level in the diagram would be likely to affect which species?

A) Spiders and toads
B) Hawks and snakes
C) Both A and B
D) Neither A nor B

31. Where is the energy content highest?

A) In grass
B) In shrews
C) In snakes
D) In toads

GO ON TO THE NEXT PAGE

32. How does the lymphatic system work with the circulatory system?

A) The circulatory system produces red blood cells for the lymphatic system.
B) Lymph draws excess fluid from the spaces between cells and deposits it into the blood vessels.
C) The heart regulates the production of lymph in the lymph glands.
D) White cells from the lymphatic system eliminate excess red blood cells.

33. The organ system primarily responsible for integrating voluntary movements is the _____ system.

Which of the following correctly completes the sentence above?

A) cardiovascular
B) digestive
C) respiratory
D) nervous

34. How do evaporation and boiling of a liquid primarily differ?

A) In speed and product
B) In temperature and speed
C) In pressure and product
D) In speed and pressure

35. A researcher looked for a correlation between children's weight and the amount of fast food they ate. The results were as follows.

Weight	87	75	68	70	94	85	90
Fast-food meals per week	0	3	2	1	4	3	1

How would you describe the correlation between weight and fast food meals per week?

A) Direct
B) Inverse
C) No correlation
D) Logarithmic

GO ON TO THE NEXT PAGE

36. In an experiment designed to examine the effects of eye makeup on women with contact lenses, which variable might be considered extraneous?

A) Age
B) Contact wearing
C) Gender
D) Use of eye makeup

37. From which part of the lungs is oxygen absorbed into the blood?

A) Bronchioles
B) Bronchi
C) Pleura
D) Alveoli

38. Which disease is most likely to result in softening of the bones?

A) Osteomyelitis
B) Lyme disease
C) Gout
D) Rickets

39. What is the main function of ribosomes?

A) Mitosis
B) Protein synthesis
C) Cellular movement
D) Storage

40. Diploid and haploid cells differ in their _____ of _____.

Which of the following correctly completes the sentence above?

A) separations; proteins
B) lengths; DNA
C) production; enzymes
D) numbers; chromosomes

41. Which might be considered a polygenic trait in humans?

A) Hair color
B) Color blindness
C) Hemophilia
D) Attached earlobes

GO ON TO THE NEXT PAGE

42. What does a pregnancy test measure?

    A) Oxytocin
    B) Progesterone
    C) Estrogen
    D) hCG

43. Dogs, goats, and pigs belong to the same

    A) species.
    B) phylum.
    C) genus.
    D) order.

44. The tonsils are part of which body system?

    A) Digestive
    B) Lymphatic
    C) Respiratory
    D) Cardiovascular

45. Which of the following may form a gallstone?

    A) Undigested food
    B) Infectious bacteria
    C) Crystallized bile
    D) Intestinal blockage

46. How are epithelial cells classified?

    A) By shape and alignment
    B) By location and function
    C) By shape and function
    D) By orientation and color

47. Which kind of immunity from disease can a baby receive through its mother's breast milk?

    A) Naturally acquired passive immunity
    B) Naturally acquired active immunity
    C) Artificially acquired passive immunity
    D) Artificially acquired active immunity

48. Which organ does *not* manufacture digestive enzymes?

    A) Kidneys
    B) Small intestine
    C) Pancreas
    D) Stomach

GO ON TO THE NEXT PAGE

49. Which parts of the heart are separated by the mitral valve?

    A) Left atrium and right atrium
    B) Right atrium and right ventricle
    C) Left ventricle and right ventricle
    D) Left atrium and left ventricle

50. In what form is glucose stored in the liver?

    A) As fatty acid
    B) As glycogen
    C) As amylase
    D) As amino acid

51. What is the function of the dendrites?

    A) Reception of stimuli
    B) Production of neurotransmitters
    C) Connection of neurons
    D) Control of sympathetic nerves

52. In which structure do sperm mature?

    A) Vas deferens
    B) Epididymis
    C) Urethra
    D) Seminiferous tubules

53. Zero population growth occurs when the numbers of births plus _____ equals the numbers of deaths plus _____.

Which of the following correctly completes the sentence above?

    A) immigrants; immigrants
    B) immigrants; emigrants
    C) emigrants; emigrants
    D) emigrants; immigrants

STOP. THIS IS THE END OF PART III.

Part IV. English and Language Usage

28 items (24 scored), 28 minutes

1. My _____ is in _____ of two tickets to the game.

   Which of the following correctly completes the sentence above?

   A) niece; reciept
   B) niece; receipt
   C) neice; reciept
   D) neice; receipt

2. Daniel is interested in the study of _____.

   Which of the following correctly completes the sentence above?

   A) sychology
   B) psycholagy
   C) psycology
   D) psychology

3. Before I had finished supper, James _____.

   Which of the following correctly completes the sentence above?

   A) is texting me on my cell phone
   B) had texted me on my cell phone
   C) texts me on my cell phone
   D) texting me on my cell phone

4. Everyone in the fraternity found the four boy's pranks sophomoric.

   What is the error in this sentence?

   A) Everyone
   B) fraternity
   C) boy's
   D) sophomoric

5. The children became bellicose after too much time in the moving car.

   What is the simple predicate of this sentence?

   A) children
   B) became
   C) after
   D) moving

GO ON TO THE NEXT PAGE

---

6. Without further ado or additional waiting, the passengers were efficiently and deferentially ushered aboard.

   Which words are redundant in the sentence above?

   A) further, ado
   B) ado, waiting
   C) further, additional
   D) efficiently, deferentially

7. Over the years, my knee joints have lost their spring.

   What is the meaning of *spring* in the sentence above?

   A) Resilience
   B) Origin
   C) Sudden jump
   D) Escape

8. Which of these sentences represents the topic sentence of a paragraph?

   A) Water from people's faucets has turned gritty and brown.
   B) We expect the mayor to call for water rationing soon.
   C) Newly planted trees are wilting and dropping leaves.
   D) The drought is causing a variety of problems in town.

9. Frederica is trying to psych herself into asking her director for a raise.

   Which word in the sentence above is slang?

   A) psych
   B) asking
   C) director
   D) raise

10. Which sentence is the clearest?

    A) In the mailbox, there was a note from her boyfriend.
    B) From her boyfriend, there was a note in the mailbox.
    C) There was in the mailbox a note from her boyfriend.
    D) In the mailbox there was from her boyfriend a note.

GO ON TO THE NEXT PAGE

11. In the apartment house, the car with the white roof and new tires belongs to our friends.

Which phrase or clause is misplaced in the sentence above?

A) In the apartment house
B) with the white roof
C) and new tires
D) to our friends

12. Which of the sentences below is most clear and correct?

A) Tapping the beat, Ms. Schuster led the chorus in song.
B) Ms. Schuster led the chorus in song tapping the beat.
C) Ms. Schuster led the chorus, tapping the beat, in song.
D) Tapping the beat, the chorus was led in song by Ms. Schuster.

13. One out of four doctors _____ to this plan.

Which of the following correctly completes the sentence above?

A) subscribe
B) subscribes
C) subscribing
D) are subscribed

14. Which sentence is the clearest?

A) A vegetable garden was planted by the family behind the house.
B) The family planted a vegetable garden behind the house.
C) The family behind the house planted a vegetable garden.
D) A vegetable garden behind the house was planted by the family.

15. With torn pages, I returned the book I'd just bought to the store.

Which phrase or clause is misplaced in the sentence above?

A) With torn pages
B) the book
C) I'd just bought
D) to the store

GO ON TO THE NEXT PAGE

16. Surprising <u>Kristina</u> a day before the holidays, Gerald presented _____ with two tickets to Aruba.

Which of the following options correctly completes the sentence? The antecedent of the pronoun to be added is underlined.

A) it
B) him
C) them
D) her

17. After waiting for Myron for nearly half an hour _____ Rochelle made a phone call and invited his twin brother to join her for dinner.

Which of the following punctuation marks correctly completes the sentence above?

A) ;
B) :
C) -
D) ,

18. The Malones told me that _____ having _____ new TV delivered this Wednesday.

Which of the following sets of words should be used to fill in the blanks in the sentence above?

A) their; there
B) there; their
C) they're; their
D) their; they're

19. When he left the army, he had achieved the rank of _____.

Which of the following is the correct completion of the sentence above?

A) luetenant
B) lieutenant
C) liutenant
D) lieutenent

20. In which word does the suffix change a verb to an adjective?

A) Dangerous
B) Rationalist
C) Agreement
D) Washable

GO ON TO THE NEXT PAGE

21. Which of the following is an example of a correctly punctuated sentence?

   A) Have you seen the fascinating television show called "Modern Life"?

   B) Have you seen the fascinating television show called "Modern Life."

   C) Have you seen the fascinating television show called "Modern Life?"

   D) Have you seen the fascinating television show called "Modern Life"!

22. The sound of the foghorn was noticed by all of us.

   Which of the following changes the sentence above so that it is written in the active rather than in the passive voice?

   A) The sound of the foghorn was heard by all of us.
   B) By all of us, the sound of the foghorn was noticed.
   C) All of us noticed the sound of the foghorn.
   D) The sound was noticed by all of us of the foghorn.

23. Which of the following sentences has correct subject-verb agreement?

   A) Donna or her sisters writes to me once a week.
   B) Neither James nor his roommate has a car.
   C) Everybody in those villages vote regularly.
   D) Few in the class has read the material yet.

24. Traffic accidents are a regular _____ along Route 5.

   Which of the following is the correct completion of the sentence above?

   A) ocurrence
   B) occurrance
   C) occurrence
   D) occurence

25. Greta <u>happily</u> followed the tennis match, her head bouncing <u>back</u> and forth.

   Which of the following correctly identifies the parts of speech in the underlined portions of the sentence above?

   A) Adverb; adjective
   B) Adjective; adverb
   C) Adjective; adjective
   D) Adverb; adverb

GO ON TO THE NEXT PAGE

26. Which of the following addresses follows the rules of capitalization?

    A) 22 west Hartford Street
    B) 14 Oak Crest place
    C) 204 Fellowship Road East
    D) 1901 southern Boulevard

27. Which of the following is an example of a simple sentence?

    A) All of my plans for the evening were no match for the formidable personality of my ancient Aunt Agnes.
    B) When Aunt Agnes arrived, my plans for the evening went right out the window.
    C) My formidable Aunt Agnes spoiled my plans for the evening; I was no match for her!
    D) I had made plans for the evening, but Aunt Agnes's arrival put an end to them.

28. Which of the following is the best definition of the word *histogenesis*?

    A) Rising blood
    B) Beginning of time
    C) Past origins
    D) Tissue growth

STOP. THIS IS THE END OF TEAS PRACTICE TEST 4.

TEAS Practice Test 4: Answer Key

PART I: READING

1. B	19. A	37. A
2. B	20. C	38. C
3. D	21. C	39. D
4. C	22. C	40. C
5. C	23. A	41. D
6. D	24. C	42. A
7. D	25. A	43. C
8. A	26. D	44. C
9. D	27. D	45. A
10. C	28. D	46. C
11. A	29. B	47. C
12. C	30. A	48. D
13. C	31. C	49. D
14. D	32. B	50. B
15. B	33. A	51. A
16. C	34. B	52. C
17. B	35. B	53. D
18. D	36. D	

PART II: MATHEMATICS

1. D	13. B	25. D
2. C	14. B	26. D
3. B	15. D	27. C
4. C	16. B	28. B
5. A	17. D	29. C
6. C	18. D	30. A
7. A	19. D	31. B
8. D	20. A	32. D
9. C	21. C	33. C
10. B	22. B	34. C
11. B	23. A	35. D
12. C	24. C	36. B

PART III: SCIENCE

1. B	19. C	37. D
2. A	20. B	38. D
3. D	21. C	39. B
4. B	22. A	40. D
5. A	23. B	41. A
6. C	24. A	42. D
7. A	25. B	43. B
8. A	26. C	44. B
9. D	27. D	45. C
10. B	28. A	46. A
11. C	29. C	47. A
12. C	30. C	48. A
13. C	31. A	49. D
14. C	32. B	50. B
15. D	33. D	51. C
16. B	34. B	52. B
17. D	35. C	53. B
18. B	36. A	

PART IV: ENGLISH AND LANGUAGE USAGE

1. B	11. A	21. A
2. D	12. A	22. C
3. B	13. B	23. B
4. C	14. B	24. C
5. B	15. A	25. D
6. C	16. D	26. C
7. A	17. D	27. A
8. D	18. C	28. D
9. A	19. B	
10. A	20. D	

TEAS Practice Test 4: Explanatory Answers

PART I: READING

1. (B) The step-by-step directions are typical of a technical manual.

2. (B) The passage tells what to do first, second, third, and so on.

3. (D) The passage instructs the reader in the steps required to perform certain tasks.

4. (C) There is no support for choice A in the passage. Since the first paragraph is about sending text messages to landlines, choice B cannot be correct. The fact that the device has more than one mode makes choice D unlikely.

5. (C) This is the sort of writing you would find in a technical manual.

6. (D) Raccoons might leave claw marks or eat seeds, but they could not bend iron bars.

7. (D) This is Pete's opinion. The other choices are facts.

8. (A) Narrative writing tells a story.

9. (D) This sentence summarizes the story by expressing a personal interpretation.

10. (C) Sharing their space with the bear is a challenge, but the author does not seem to find it annoying (choice D) or scary (choices A and B).

11. (A) Nature is a theme of the passage; the topic is getting visits from a bear.

12. (C) The three short paragraphs are entertaining when put together; they show Pete's movement from denial to acceptance.

13. (C) It is too late to put on protective gear (choice A). Testing the blade while it is spinning is surely a bad idea (choice B). The wood is cut, so avoiding the burls should have taken place earlier (choice D).

14. (D) The directions tell how to use this particular kind of saw.

15. (B) To find a list of chapters, look in the table of contents.

16. (C) Draw a picture if it helps. Call Andy A, Bret B, Carrie C, and Dave D.

    Step 1: A B C D

    Step 2: A B D C

    Step 3: A D B C

    Step 4: D B C A

17. (B) The clue is in this sentence: "This training program will focus on the skills necessary for mid- to upper-level support positions such as Administrative Assistant, Executive Secretary, Legal Secretary, and Medical Secretary." A secretary already versed in these skills will not benefit (choice C), and the course is not designed for nurses (choice A) or administrators (choice D).

18. (D) *Nebulous* is related to *nebula*, meaning "cloud." A nebulous answer is cloudy, or vague.

19. (A) Enviro-Control seems to be a place that does environmental testing.

20. (C) Kiowa Medical Center is listed with a main site and a branch site at the mall.

21. (C) Pounds are listed clockwise around the outside of the scale. The highest value labeled is 280, but the scale extends a bit above that.

22. (C) The label indicates that this product has 3 percent of the daily requirement of sodium (choice A), 2 percent calcium (choice B), and 0 percent vitamin C (choice D). However, it does have 23 percent of the daily requirement for cholesterol.

23. (A) The gingival margin is the edge of the gums.

24. (C) The directions state that waiting longer will not strengthen the anesthetic effect (choice A), that the effect lasts about 20 minutes (making choice B unlikely), and that the gel may be reapplied (choice D). Apparently, waiting to begin simply wastes part of the 20-minute window.

25. (A) The author states some effects first in the form of symptoms before naming the cause—reduced amounts of hypocretin.

26. (D) Laughing too hard and its subsequent effect are simply supporting details in the overall description of narcolepsy.

27. (D) The would-be seller might place an ad in the classified section.

28. (D) Stella travels eight stops on the local line. Della travels three stops on the express line, or five fewer than Stella.

29. (B) There is only one local stop that meets these parameters—the one south of the museum. The man must transfer to the express stop at the museum and then travel west one express stop to end at the mall.

30. (A) Odysseus was a Greek hero, but he was not a god.

31. (C) First look for the stores that carry floral comforters: choices A, B, and C. Then look for those that carry queen sizes: choices B and C. Finally find the one that is under $100: choice C.

32. (B) A road map (choice A) does not have the scale required, and a travel brochure (choice C) is also fairly limited in scope. The best choice is a world atlas (choice B), which allows the traveler to see the entire world of possibilities.

33. (A) "Appetite control" and "appetite suppressants" may fit under the topic of diet and nutrition. Since they are on pages 187 and 181, the chapter must encompass those pages.

34. (B) Moving section 1 to the right gives you section 2 stacked atop section 3 with section 1 along the right edge of each. Then rotating that shape to the left (counterclockwise) gives you a shape with section 1 on top, section 2 on the left, and section 3 on the right.

35. (B) A positive connotation is an affirmative feeling attached to a word, separate from its dictionary definition. In this case, choices A, C, and D all hint at the spendthrift quality of the banquet—the extreme nature of the event. Only choice B manages to describe its abundance without being negative.

36. (D) The list must contain proper adjectives related to countries in Europe. Only choice D follows this rule.

37. (A) If the trainers are accredited, they have credentials proving their qualifications.

38. (C) The writer encourages people to take advantage of the training, implying that he thinks it is worthwhile.

39. (D) The author speaks of women's dependence on men as retarding their moral growth.

40. (C) Writings from all parts of history might deal with questions of morality (B), but only at a certain point in time did writers expound on the restrictiveness of women's lives.

41. (D) Imagine four towns laid out from west to east, with 5-mile intervals between them:

Daly   Compton   Barnard   Addison

The problem really begins with step 5. The train, beginning in Daly, travels back and forth for 30 miles: 5 to Compton, 5 more to Barnard, 5 more to Addison, 5 more to Barnard, 5 more to Compton, and 5 more to Daly again.

42. (A) The first website is the only one that mentions causes, so it is probably the one to turn to first.

43. (C) Degrees Fahrenheit are on the right side of this thermometer. The column indicates a temperature of about 76 degrees Fahrenheit.

44. (C) Feathered Friends' and Birdland's deals are the simplest, so go there first. Feathered Friends' cost is $30. Birdland's is $22 + $5, or $27. It should be clear without doing the math that no one's deal will beat Birdland's.

45. (A) Jason can buy four bags for $100 if the bags cost $25 apiece or less. That makes Pets & More and Birdland his only possible choices.

46. (C) Find the bars for 1960 and then compare. New York's population was nearly 8 million. Philadelphia's was about 2 million. The best answer is choice C.

47. (C) To answer this, compare all four of the light-colored bars. The bar for 1960 is longest.

48. (D) *Repair* has many meanings, but only this one fits the context of the sentence.

49. (D) The author's argument is that vinegar kills weeds "without harming anything else." If it in fact kills other plants besides weeds, that contradicts the argument.

50. (B) The conclusion must follow directly from the argument. The passage says that "vinegar is an effective and risk-free weed killer," meaning that by using vinegar, a homeowner may avoid using toxic chemicals to kill weeds. Choice A is negated by the passage, choice C may be true but is not part of the passage, and choice D is suggested but is not well supported.

51. (A) Another way to think of the sentence is: *Even though Doris had not yet received her degree, her advisor encouraged her to apply to the prestigious graduate program.* The word that best expresses this contrast is choice A, *nevertheless*.

52. (C) Only this choice can be proved or checked. The other choices express opinions, as indicated by words such as *dangerous, mild, nasty*, and *should*.

53. (D) *Hazardous waste* is a label placed on the bin. This is an example of words used as words, a typical reason for the use of italics.

Part II: Mathematics

1. (D) Decimals are expressed as tenths, hundredths, and so on. Think: $\frac{9}{25} \times \frac{4}{4} = \frac{36}{100}$. The decimal equivalent is 0.36.

2. (C) There are several steps to this problem. The posts average 5 feet, or 60 inches, tall. Farmer Brown wants 52-inch posts. He cuts 6 inches off three posts to get them to 52 inches, which means that they were 58 inches to start with. Now you have enough information to determine the height of the fourth post: $\frac{(58 + 58 + 58 + x)}{4} = 60$. Solve: $\frac{(174 + x)}{4} = 60$, so $(174 + x) = 240$. $x = 240 - 174$, or 66 inches tall. To get that fourth post down to 52 inches, Farmer Brown must hack off 14 inches.

3. (B) The paperbacks cost 0.35×5, or $1.75. The hardcover books cost 2.50×3, or $7.50. Together, they cost $1.75 + $7.50, or $9.25. Subtract that from $10 to find the change: $10.00 - $9.25 = $0.75.

4. (C) Ordinarily, multiplying two numbers with two digits right of the decimal point would result in a product with four digits to the right of the decimal point. Here, however, the last digit, zero, is dropped off.

5. (A) If 2.2 pounds = 1 kilogram, 11 pounds = $\frac{11}{2.2}$ kilograms, or 5 kilograms.

6. (C) Think of this as a proportion: $\frac{3 \text{ bars}}{\$2.58} = 5$ bars/x. Cross-multiply to solve: $5(\$2.58) = 3x$, so $\$12.90 = 3x$, so $\$4.30 = x$. You may also solve this by figuring out the unit cost: $\frac{\$2.58}{3} = \$0.86$ per bar, so 5 bars would cost $\$0.86 \times 5 = \$4.30$.

7. (A) Solve by dividing Clara's homes by the total and expressing the resulting decimal as a percent. $244 \div 1{,}525 = 0.16$, or 16%.

8. (D) Multiply the unknowns first: $2x \times 2x = 4x^2$. Then multiply $2x \times -2$ and $2x \times 2$, for a total of $-4x + 4x$, or 0. Finally, multiply -2×2.

9. (C) The perimeter is the distance around the field, so it is 25 yards + 40 yards + 25 yards + 40 yards, or 130 yards.

10. (B) You barely need to compute here; you just must read the graph. On Friday, Beantown Library checked out around 84 books, and Teeburg Library checked out around 72, for a difference of 12 books.

11. (B) In 1950, you could buy gas for 26.4¢ per gallon. Divide that into $5.00, remembering to express cents as part of a dollar, to find the greatest number of gallons you could have purchased for $5.00: $\$5.00 \div \$0.264 = 18.93939$. The greatest number of gallons would have been 18.

12. (C) If you remember that dividing by a fraction is the same as multiplying by its reciprocal, you needn't bother to do the computation here. $4\frac{1}{8} \div \frac{1}{4}$ is the same as $4\frac{1}{8} \times 4$, which is close to 16. Check by doing the math: $\frac{33}{8} \times \frac{4}{1} = \frac{132}{8} = 16\frac{4}{8}$, or $16\frac{1}{2}$.

13. (B) The median cost is the one in the middle—half are greater, and half are less.

14. (B) Since you are multiplying a number with two digits after the decimal point by a number with one digit after the decimal point, the answer should have three digits after the decimal point.

15. (D) 1,000 grams = 1 kilogram, so 14,000 grams = 14 kilograms.

16. (B) Texas is still growing, as are California and Florida, but New York is standing still. That makes choice B the only logical forecast.

17. (D) If 1 knot = 1.852 kph, 25 knots = 1.852×25, or 46.3 kph. The wind speed was under that level for all five days shown.

18. (D) Express the mixed number as an improper fraction: $\frac{17}{3}$. Then find the lowest common denominator and restate the two fractions: $\frac{119}{21} + \frac{18}{21}$. Solve, and express as a mixed number in lowest terms: $\frac{137}{21} = 6\frac{11}{21}$.

19. (D) $6 + 6 = 12$, $12 + 30 = 42$, and $42 - 2 = 40$.

20. (A) The dependent variable is the one whose changes depend on the independent variable. In this case, hatching depends on time.

21. (C) The answer will be close to but not greater than 8, since $8^2 = 64$. Test the two closest numbers that are less than 8: $7.75 \times 7.75 = 60.0625$, and $7.95 \times 7.95 = 63.2025$. 7.95 is closer.

22. (B) Each carton cost nearly $25. $25 × 12 = $300. That is close to the actual cost: $24.95 × 12 = $299.40.

23. (A) Express the mixed numbers as improper fractions, and then multiply numerators and denominators. $4\frac{5}{6} = \frac{29}{6} \cdot 1\frac{1}{8} = \frac{9}{8} \cdot \frac{29}{6} \times \frac{9}{8} = \frac{261}{48}$. Now express the answer as a mixed number in lowest terms. $\frac{261}{48} = 5\frac{21}{48}$, or $5\frac{7}{16}$.

24. (C) Al began with $1,280.75 and over the course of the month added $989.25 and $989.25, for a total of $3,259.25. He took out $20 + $50 + $675 + $50 + $25.30, or $820.30 in all. Subtract that from his income to find his balance at the end of the month: $3,259.25 − $820.30 = $2,438.95.

25. (D) Use common sense. The first number is a bit more than 5. The second is a bit more than 2. Multiplying them must give you a product that is greater than 10.

26. (D) Put this into an equation: $\frac{(2.8 \text{ kg} + 3.8 \text{ kg} + 2.9 \text{ kg} + 3.1 \text{ kg} + x)}{5} = $ 3.2 kg. Multiply both sides by 5 to get (2.8 kg + 3.8 kg + 2.9 kg + 3.1 kg + x) = 16 kg. Perform the addition: (12.6 kg + x) = 16 kg; so x = 3.4 kg.

27. (C) You know that 100% of 75 = 75, so 125% must be greater, and choices A and B are clearly incorrect. 1.25(75) = 93.75.

28. (B) The units don't matter here; the scale is 2:1. If 2 cm = 1 m, 8 cm = 4 m, and 10 cm = 5 m.

29. (C) The dosage is small, so the tool should be small as well.

30. (A) Read this as "the absolute value of negative 2 times the absolute value of 3." Absolute value is always a positive number.

31. (B) Twice John's nephew's height is 2c, and 20 less than that is 2c − 20. Suppose the nephew's height is 48 inches. John's is 96 − 20 inches, or 76 inches.

32. (D) −17.5 is less than −17. $\frac{34}{2} = 17$. The least number in the list is −17.5, and the greatest is $\frac{34}{2}$.

33. (C) Circle graphs are good for comparing percentages.

34. (C) Choice A would earn 7 + 9, or 16 points. Choice B would earn 14 + 3, or 17 points, to tie the game. Choice D would earn 21 points, which would win, but not by the minimum number of points. That minimum is represented by choice C, which earns 14 + 6, or 20 points in all.

35. (D) No real pattern is discernible in these data points, meaning that there is no obvious correlation between the *x* and *y* values.

36. (B) Plain cones would be $2x—each cone would cost $2, and the total number of plain cones would be represented by *x*. Cones with sprinkles cost 50 cents more, so they would be $2.5y, with each cone costing $2.50 and the total number of cones with sprinkles represented by *y*. To find how much the father paid, you need to add both expressions, as in choice B.

Part III: Science

1. (B) The skull surrounds the brain, making it superficial, or closer to the body surface.

2. (A) A sagittal section occurs along a longitudinal plane, dividing the body into right and left regions.

3. (D) In the final step of an experiment, you develop a conclusion and suggest where to go next.

4. (B) The esophagus is the passage that connects the pharynx to the stomach.

5. (A) The sympathetic and parasympathetic systems (choices C and D) are part of the autonomic nervous system (choice B), which controls involuntary actions of the smooth muscles, glands, and heart. The somatic nervous system (choice A) has to do with reception of external stimuli and voluntary control of the muscles.

6. (C) Damage to a disc in the lower back will most likely cause pain radiating downward along the sciatic nerve.

7. (A) *Empirical* means "based on experiment and observation rather than theory."

8. (A) Reading the chart clockwise from top left, the cross would yield one female carrier, one female hemophiliac, one male hemophiliac, and one normal male who neither carries nor manifests the disease.

9. (D) At point X, transcription is "unzipping" DNA to form a strand of mRNA. The mRNA then creates a protein through translation, as shown at Y.

10. (B) The log phase is a phase of exponential growth.

11. (C) This choice reduces the possibility that one brand might emit more radiation than another; it also allows for a before-and-after measurement that is parallel for each test.

12. (C) Leaving the bottles in sunlight for equal amounts of time would determine whether solar power disinfected them differently. Step A is already done; step D should be done after C is complete; and step B does not contribute to a testing of the hypothesis.

13. (C) Meiosis is the cell division that results in reproductive cells. Meiosis I results in the creation of two daughter cells, each containing half the chromosomes of the parent cell. Meiosis II continues through a process similar to mitosis, resulting in four daughter cells, each with half the chromosomes of the parent cell.

14. (C) Thiamine (B_1) deficiency is often found in people whose diet consists largely of polished white rice; in refining the rice, the thiamine-rich husk is removed. Beriberi may affect several systems in the body and may lead to paralysis or death.

15. (D) Diuretics eliminate water from the system, sometimes causing electrolyte imbalance and a drop in blood pressure. They do not address the causes of obesity, and their effects last only a short while.

16. (B) Ice (choice D) floats on water (choice B) because its density is less, despite the fact that it is a solid. When water freezes, its volume increases, making its density (mass/volume) less.

17. (D) The gas with the least mass will diffuse most rapidly.

18. (B) The cerebellum, located at the back of the skull, coordinates muscle activity and controls balance, posture, voluntary movement, and adaptive motor skills.

19. (C) The normal range of urine output is 800 mL to 2 L per day. Polyuria, or excessive urination, is diagnosed when output exceeds 2.5 L daily.

20. (B) Stem cells produced in the bone marrow may stay there to mature into B cells or migrate to the thymus gland to mature into T cells. Until they mature either as helper or cytoxic T cells, they are known as thymocytes.

21. (C) The atomic number of an element equals the number of protons in its nucleus. Of the numbers given, only 11, Na (sodium), is an alkali metal.

22. (A) Line I indicates a species that survives well through the early part of its expected life span and only dies off in large numbers toward the end. This would be typical of humans or other species that have few offspring, which are cared for by adults immediately after birth and for a while thereafter.

23. (B) Notice where the 0 is on the *y*-axis. The collapse of species appears to be most rapid in low-diversity regions.

24. (A) Again, notice where the 0 is on the *y*-axis. Decline of species increases over time, making this a direct correlation.

25. (B) Loose irregular tissue (choice C) might be found in a lymph gland. It contains a loose arrangement of fibers and a variety of cells in fluid. Dense irregular tissue (choice D) is more tightly woven and may be found in the dermis, among other sites. Dense regular tissue (choice B) is specialized connective tissue found in tendons and ligaments. In this kind of tissue, collagen fibers are densely packed and aligned. Only dense connective tissue is identified as regular or irregular, making choice A impossible.

26. (C) Acid + base $\rightarrow$ salt + water.

27. (D) The epidermis ranges from about 0.05 mm thick on the eyelid to around 1.5 mm thick on the palm of the hand and sole of the foot.

28. (A) A higher concentration of sweat glands exists in the feet than anywhere else in the body. The back (choice C) actually has a very low concentration of glands. Eccrine sweat glands secrete mainly water and salt. Apocrine sweat glands, which secrete a combination of lipids, steroids, and proteins, are mainly in the armpits, genitals, breasts, and ear canals. These are the secretions that have an odor when they meet with bacteria and begin to break down.

29. (C) The spleen is a fist-shaped organ to the left of the stomach in the upper left section of the abdomen.

30. (C) The second trophic level on the diagram includes every primary consumer that eats grass—the shrew, the groundhog, and the locust. Such a die-out would affect everything that eats animals at that level, including the spider, toad, hawk, and garter snake.

31. (A) Energy is always highest in producers and dissipates up the food chain.

32. (B) One of the jobs of the lymphatic system is to prevent excess fluid from accumulating in tissues by collecting it and moving it into the circulatory system via the brachiocephalic veins.

33. (D) The nervous system controls the voluntary movements of the skeletal system.

34. (B) Evaporation is a vaporization that happens slowly across the surface of a liquid. It can occur at any temperature. Boiling, on the other hand, occurs rapidly throughout a liquid when the temperature of the liquid reaches its boiling point.

35. (C) If you were to graph these results, you would see little or no pattern, meaning that there is no correlation.

36. (A) The experiment relies on contact-wearing women who wear eye makeup. Age is never specified.

37. (D) The alveoli are the site of gas exchange in the lungs. They are tiny, balloon-like structures that terminate each branch of the bronchial passages.

38. (D) All of the diseases listed may affect bone tissue, but only rickets, caused by a vitamin D deficiency, is characterized by a softening of the bones.

39. (B) Ribosomes translate mRNA to manufacture protein from amino acids.

40. (D) Diploid cells have two sets of chromosomes; haploid cells have only one.

41. (A) A polygenic trait is controlled by more than one gene. Choices B, C, and D do not fit into that category.

42. (D) Human chorionic gonadotropin (hCG) is produced by what will become the placenta. If pregnancy occurs, the level of hCG rises exponentially, starting immediately upon the egg's implantation in the uterus. The level of hCG may be measured by a blood or urine test.

43. (B) Dogs, goats, and pigs all have backbones, and thus are in the phylum Chordata. Dogs are in the order Carnivora, but goats and pigs are not. Both are Artiodactyla (even-toed ungulates).

44. (B) The tonsils are clusters of lymphatic cells located in the pharynx. Their function is to defend against inhaled or ingested pathogens.

45. (C) The gallbladder stores bile from the liver, but occasionally, the bile from the liver has excess cholesterol, excess bilirubin, or not enough bile salts. In such cases, the bile can form crystals, which may clump together and block one of the bile ducts.

46. (A) Epithelial cells come in different shapes and are arranged in strata one or more cells thick. Examples of classifications might be "simple cuboidal," "simple columnar," or "stratified squamous."

47. (A) Breast milk transfers certain antibodies from the mother to the infant.

48. (A) The small intestine (choice B) manufactures maltase and peptidase; the pancreas (choice C) manufactures pancreatic amylase, trypsin, and lipase; and the stomach (choice D) manufactures pepsin.

49. (D) The mitral valve opens to allow oxygenated blood collected in the left atrium to flow into the left ventricle.

50. (B) The liver converts glucose to glycogen and stores it, keeping blood sugar levels balanced.

51. (C) *Dendrites*, from the Greek word for "trees," branch off of neurons and help connect one neuron to the next via synapses.

52. (B) Sperm cells are manufactured in the seminiferous tubules (choice D) of the testes and stored in the narrow tube called the epididymis (choice B) until ejaculated via the vas deferens and urethra (choices A and C).

53. (B) Population growth involves both birth and immigration; population decline involves both death and emigration.

Part IV: English and Language Usage

1. (B) The two words follow the rule "*i* before *e*, except after *c*."

2. (D) Dividing the word into its roots—*psych* + *ology*—may help you spell it correctly.

3. (B) The verbs in the sentence must be parallel.

4. (C) If there are four boys, the possessive noun that refers to them all must be *boys'*, with an apostrophe after the plural noun.

5. (B) The predicate is the verb; in this case, *became* (choice B).

6. (C) Only *further* and *additional* are synonymous and can be considered redundant, or repetitive.

7. (A) In this context, *spring* refers to the elasticity of the knee joints, making *resilience* the best synonym.

8. (D) The topic sentence should introduce the topic or key idea. In this case, the order of sentences in the paragraph might logically be D, A, C, B. Choice D is the topic sentence, because it introduces the drought. Choices A and C add supporting details about the problems caused by the drought, and choice B provides a conclusion that makes a prediction about what might come next.

9. (A) To *psych* or *psych up* is a slang term meaning "to prepare mentally."

10. (A) If in doubt, read the sentences aloud and pick the one that is least convoluted.

11. (A) The car is not in the apartment house; the friends are. Moving the phrase *in the apartment house* to the end of the sentence would improve the logic of the sentence.

12. (A) Ms. Schuster is the one tapping the beat, so the modifying phrase should be as close as possible to her name.

13. (B) The subject of the sentence is *one*, so the verb should be singular.

14. (B) Was the family behind the house? No, the garden was. Choice B offers the best, most logical construction.

15. (A) I did not have torn pages; my book did. Placing the phrase closer to the word it modifies would improve the sentence.

16. (D) *Kristina* is both singular and feminine, making *her* the only possible choice.

17. (D) *After waiting for Myron for nearly half an hour* is a phrase, not a clause (it does not contain a subject and verb combination). Therefore, it requires a comma to separate it from the rest of the sentence, not a semicolon (choice A).

18. (C) *They're* means "they are," *their* means "belonging to them," and *there* means "in that place."

19. (B) A *lieutenant* is an officer who serves in place of a superior at certain times. For that reason, the title means "place" (*lieu*) "holder" (*tenant*).

20. (D) Although *dangerous* is an adjective (choice A), the suffix *-ous* changes a noun to an adjective, not a verb to an adjective, as in choice D. In choice B, the suffix changes an adjective to a noun. In choice C, the suffix changes a verb to a noun. Choice D takes the verb *wash* and makes it into an adjective meaning "able to be washed."

21. (A) The question mark is not part of the television show's title; it is part of the sentence as a whole. For that reason, it belongs outside the quotation marks.

22. (C) To make this passive sentence active, you must remove the subject from the prepositional phrase and connect it to the action of the verb.

23. (B) In sentences having a compound subject with *or* (choice A), the verb must agree with the closest noun or pronoun, in this case, *sisters*. *Everybody* (choice C) is always singular, and *few* (choice D) is always plural.

24. (C) Only choice C is a word. The rule is: Double the final consonant in *occur* and add the suffix. However, knowing whether to add *–ence* or *–ance* is a matter of memorization.

25. (D) *Happily* tells how Greta followed the match, and *back* tells where her head bounced. Both modify verbs, so both are adverbs.

26. (C) All names of streets must be capitalized, including direction words within the names.

27. (A) A simple sentence may have a compound subject or a compound predicate, but it will never have two separate subject and predicate combinations. Sentence B is complex; it contains a dependent clause and an independent clause. Both sentences C and D contain two independent clauses.

28. (D) *Histo-* means "tissue," and *genesis* means "creation" or "evolution."

TEAS PRACTICE TEST 5

TEAS Practice Test 5: Answer Sheet

READING

1 (A) (B) (C) (D)	19 (A) (B) (C) (D)	37 (A) (B) (C) (D)
2 (A) (B) (C) (D)	20 (A) (B) (C) (D)	38 (A) (B) (C) (D)
3 (A) (B) (C) (D)	21 (A) (B) (C) (D)	39 (A) (B) (C) (D)
4 (A) (B) (C) (D)	22 (A) (B) (C) (D)	40 (A) (B) (C) (D)
5 (A) (B) (C) (D)	23 (A) (B) (C) (D)	41 (A) (B) (C) (D)
6 (A) (B) (C) (D)	24 (A) (B) (C) (D)	42 (A) (B) (C) (D)
7 (A) (B) (C) (D)	25 (A) (B) (C) (D)	43 (A) (B) (C) (D)
8 (A) (B) (C) (D)	26 (A) (B) (C) (D)	44 (A) (B) (C) (D)
9 (A) (B) (C) (D)	27 (A) (B) (C) (D)	45 (A) (B) (C) (D)
10 (A) (B) (C) (D)	28 (A) (B) (C) (D)	46 (A) (B) (C) (D)
11 (A) (B) (C) (D)	29 (A) (B) (C) (D)	47 (A) (B) (C) (D)
12 (A) (B) (C) (D)	30 (A) (B) (C) (D)	48 (A) (B) (C) (D)
13 (A) (B) (C) (D)	31 (A) (B) (C) (D)	49 (A) (B) (C) (D)
14 (A) (B) (C) (D)	32 (A) (B) (C) (D)	50 (A) (B) (C) (D)
15 (A) (B) (C) (D)	33 (A) (B) (C) (D)	51 (A) (B) (C) (D)
16 (A) (B) (C) (D)	34 (A) (B) (C) (D)	52 (A) (B) (C) (D)
17 (A) (B) (C) (D)	35 (A) (B) (C) (D)	53 (A) (B) (C) (D)
18 (A) (B) (C) (D)	36 (A) (B) (C) (D)	

MATHEMATICS

1 (A) (B) (C) (D)	13 (A) (B) (C) (D)	25 (A) (B) (C) (D)
2 (A) (B) (C) (D)	14 (A) (B) (C) (D)	26 (A) (B) (C) (D)
3 (A) (B) (C) (D)	15 (A) (B) (C) (D)	27 (A) (B) (C) (D)
4 (A) (B) (C) (D)	16 (A) (B) (C) (D)	28 (A) (B) (C) (D)
5 (A) (B) (C) (D)	17 (A) (B) (C) (D)	29 (A) (B) (C) (D)
6 (A) (B) (C) (D)	18 (A) (B) (C) (D)	30 (A) (B) (C) (D)
7 (A) (B) (C) (D)	19 (A) (B) (C) (D)	31 (A) (B) (C) (D)
8 (A) (B) (C) (D)	20 (A) (B) (C) (D)	32 (A) (B) (C) (D)
9 (A) (B) (C) (D)	21 (A) (B) (C) (D)	33 (A) (B) (C) (D)
10 (A) (B) (C) (D)	22 (A) (B) (C) (D)	34 (A) (B) (C) (D)
11 (A) (B) (C) (D)	23 (A) (B) (C) (D)	35 (A) (B) (C) (D)
12 (A) (B) (C) (D)	24 (A) (B) (C) (D)	36 (A) (B) (C) (D)

SCIENCE

1 (A) (B) (C) (D)   19 (A) (B) (C) (D)   37 (A) (B) (C) (D)
2 (A) (B) (C) (D)   20 (A) (B) (C) (D)   38 (A) (B) (C) (D)
3 (A) (B) (C) (D)   21 (A) (B) (C) (D)   39 (A) (B) (C) (D)
4 (A) (B) (C) (D)   22 (A) (B) (C) (D)   40 (A) (B) (C) (D)
5 (A) (B) (C) (D)   23 (A) (B) (C) (D)   41 (A) (B) (C) (D)
6 (A) (B) (C) (D)   24 (A) (B) (C) (D)   42 (A) (B) (C) (D)
7 (A) (B) (C) (D)   25 (A) (B) (C) (D)   43 (A) (B) (C) (D)
8 (A) (B) (C) (D)   26 (A) (B) (C) (D)   44 (A) (B) (C) (D)
9 (A) (B) (C) (D)   27 (A) (B) (C) (D)   45 (A) (B) (C) (D)
10 (A) (B) (C) (D)   28 (A) (B) (C) (D)   46 (A) (B) (C) (D)
11 (A) (B) (C) (D)   29 (A) (B) (C) (D)   47 (A) (B) (C) (D)
12 (A) (B) (C) (D)   30 (A) (B) (C) (D)   48 (A) (B) (C) (D)
13 (A) (B) (C) (D)   31 (A) (B) (C) (D)   49 (A) (B) (C) (D)
14 (A) (B) (C) (D)   32 (A) (B) (C) (D)   50 (A) (B) (C) (D)
15 (A) (B) (C) (D)   33 (A) (B) (C) (D)   51 (A) (B) (C) (D)
16 (A) (B) (C) (D)   34 (A) (B) (C) (D)   52 (A) (B) (C) (D)
17 (A) (B) (C) (D)   35 (A) (B) (C) (D)   53 (A) (B) (C) (D)
18 (A) (B) (C) (D)   36 (A) (B) (C) (D)

ENGLISH AND LANGUAGE USAGE

1 (A) (B) (C) (D)   11 (A) (B) (C) (D)   21 (A) (B) (C) (D)
2 (A) (B) (C) (D)   12 (A) (B) (C) (D)   22 (A) (B) (C) (D)
3 (A) (B) (C) (D)   13 (A) (B) (C) (D)   23 (A) (B) (C) (D)
4 (A) (B) (C) (D)   14 (A) (B) (C) (D)   24 (A) (B) (C) (D)
5 (A) (B) (C) (D)   15 (A) (B) (C) (D)   25 (A) (B) (C) (D)
6 (A) (B) (C) (D)   16 (A) (B) (C) (D)   26 (A) (B) (C) (D)
7 (A) (B) (C) (D)   17 (A) (B) (C) (D)   27 (A) (B) (C) (D)
8 (A) (B) (C) (D)   18 (A) (B) (C) (D)   28 (A) (B) (C) (D)
9 (A) (B) (C) (D)   19 (A) (B) (C) (D)
10 (A) (B) (C) (D)   20 (A) (B) (C) (D)

Part I. Reading

53 questions (47 scored), 64 minutes

Proposed Development Blocked

The planned apartment complex in the hamlet of Virgule ran into a snag Wednesday when residents of the hamlet came out en masse to protest it. Would-be landlord Steven Lister was taken aback at the level of concern. He promised to return with his lawyer to the next meeting of the Zoning Board of Appeals.

The development has reached this impasse because the area is zoned for no more than 10 units per acre. The Lister development calls for 15. Because the Town Board turned down the plan, Lister has turned to the Zoning Board of Appeals. In the meantime, residents up and down the valley have taken up the cause.

"We want to keep this kind of development from taking over our hamlet," explained Hector Alvarez, whose property would border the proposed apartment complex. "Adding this much population all at once puts a burden on our sewer and water plant, and it has a big impact on our roads. We estimate that traffic during rush hour will double once all of the units are occupied."

Lister is already in trouble with one resident for being a bad neighbor. "His taxes on the other apartment buildings he owns are always in arrears," says business owner Margo Shaw of Virgule Road. "Another Lister development does our town no good at all." Lister had trouble renting all of the units in his most recent development and admits that he "temporarily" fell behind on his obligations to the town. He points to improved demographics as the reason his new plan will succeed where his last one did not.

Members of the Zoning Board of Appeals have placed the Lister development first on their January agenda. Board Chair Rita Dunlap says that they hope to resolve the issue next month and move on to other things. Alvarez, Shaw, and other local residents have vowed to attend that meeting with charts and statistics in hand.

The next seven questions are based on this passage.

1. "The development has reached this impasse because the area is zoned for no more than 10 units per acre."

   The sentence above is the first sentence in the second paragraph. Related to the passage as a whole, this sentence is best described as which of the following?

   A) Main idea
   B) Topic
   C) Theme
   D) Supporting detail

GO ON TO THE NEXT PAGE

2. Which of the following is the author's main purpose for writing this article?

A) To express an opinion about excessive development in neighborhoods
B) To alert and inform residents about a controversial issue in their community
C) To compare and contrast development issues in a variety of contexts
D) To relate a story of one neighborhood's solution to an existing problem

3. Based on the passage, which conclusion can you most readily draw?

A) Lister will easily get his development approved.
B) Lister will face opposition at the next board meeting.
C) Lister will move his development to a different site.
D) Lister will join forces with the townspeople.

4. Which of the following sentences expresses the opinion of the writer or speaker?

A) Members of the Zoning Board of Appeals have placed the Lister development first on their January agenda.
B) He promised to return with his lawyer to the next meeting of the Zoning Board of Appeals.
C) "His taxes on the other apartment buildings he owns are always in arrears."
D) "Another Lister development does our town no good at all."

5. Based on the passage, you can conclude that Lister was

A) surprised at the level of concern.
B) amused at the turnout of citizens.
C) not fazed by the comments of villagers.
D) eager to make changes to his plans.

6. The passage is reflective of which of the following types of writing?

A) Narrative
B) Expository
C) Technical
D) Persuasive

GO ON TO THE NEXT PAGE

7. Which of the following sentences is the topic sentence for the entire passage?

A) The planned apartment complex in the hamlet of Virgule ran into a snag Wednesday when residents of the hamlet came out en masse to protest it.

B) Board Chair Rita Dunlap says that they hope to resolve the issue next month and move on to other things.

C) Because the Town Board turned down the plan, Lister has turned to the Zoning Board of Appeals.

D) He points to improved demographics as the reason his new plan will succeed where his last one did not.

Chalmette Battlefield

Historians consider General Andrew Jackson's victory over the British at the Battle of New Orleans the greatest land victory of the War of 1812. The victory ensured America's sovereignty over the Louisiana Territory, which in turn led to a wave of new settlement in that area.

Today the battlefield is preserved as a tourist attraction. It features a monument whose cornerstone was laid in 1840 after Jackson visited the field on the 25th anniversary of the battle. The Chalmette National Cemetery is also on the site. It houses the remains of only one veteran of the Battle of New Orleans; it is mainly for veterans of the Civil War (on the Union side), the Spanish-American War, World Wars I and II, and the Vietnam conflict.

Like all good historical restorations and most of our national historical parks, this one conjures up the history it celebrates. Visitors to the site may gain a panoramic view of the field of battle, with large reproductions of American cannons still fixed at several batteries, and the front lines clearly visible. On the left, tourists may envision Colonel Robert Rennie's attack, which briefly overtook the American rampart. In the center, small-arms fire tore through the British Highlanders troops. On the right, the brigade run by General Samuel Gibbs came to grief under fire from General John Coffee's Tennessean troops.

The next five questions are based on this passage.

8. Which of the following is the author's main purpose for writing this passage?

A) To compare Chalmette Battlefield to other great historical sites
B) To describe an interesting national historical park
C) To persuade visitors to help preserve the Chalmette Battlefield
D) To inform the reader of several key battles in the War of 1812

GO ON TO THE NEXT PAGE

9. Which of the following conclusions may be drawn directly from the first paragraph of the passage?

A) Had the battle been lost, America might have lost the Louisiana Territory.
B) Americans did not move into the Louisiana Territory before the battle.
C) Andrew Jackson was an early settler in the Louisiana Territory.
D) Most early inhabitants of the Louisiana Territory were British.

10. The passage is reflective of which of the following types of writing?

A) Narrative
B) Expository
C) Technical
D) Persuasive

11. Based on the passage, which of the following is the most likely inference?

A) The author believes that reconstructed historical sites serve no purpose.
B) The author believes that American battlegrounds are especially haunting.
C) The author believes that historical sites should help visitors imagine their history.
D) The author believes that the Chalmette Cemetery should hold only War of 1812 veterans.

12. The author's description of the battlefield in the third paragraph is reflective of which of the following types of text structure?

A) Problem-solution
B) Cause-effect
C) Chronological
D) Space order

GO ON TO THE NEXT PAGE

Directions: This vaccine must only be used <u>intramuscularly</u> and as a single dose vial. The vaccine contains no preservative or stabilizer. It should be used immediately after reconstitution, and if it is not administered promptly, discard the contents. Attach the plunger and reconstitution needle to the syringe and reconstitute the freeze-dried vaccine by injecting the diluent into the vaccine vial. Gently swirl the contents until completely dissolved and withdraw the total contents of the vial into the syringe.

The next two questions are based on this passage.

13. *Intramuscularly* means

    A) between muscles.
    B) into muscles.
    C) without muscles.
    D) on top of muscles.

14. Why must the product be used right away?

    A) It is useful only in the first hours of infection.
    B) It contains only a single dose.
    C) It functions best in the early part of the day.
    D) It can go bad or lose strength.

Some people linger in your memory far longer than you ever actually knew them in person. For me, Lindy Barker was just such a person. Even today, when I read the word *joyful*, it is Lindy's freckled face that appears before my eyes.

The next two questions are based on this passage.

15. Is the following a topic, main idea, theme, or supporting detail of the passage?

Memory

    A) Topic
    B) Main idea
    C) Theme
    D) Supporting details

16. What is the author's apparent purpose for writing this paragraph about Lindy Barker?

    A) To inform
    B) To persuade
    C) To explain
    D) To reflect

GO ON TO THE NEXT PAGE

Nutrition Facts

Serving size 1 muffin (86 g)
Servings per container 12

Amount per serving

Calories 170	Calories from fat 5

	% Daily value*
Total fat 1 g	1%
Saturated fat 0 g	0%
Trans fat 0 g	
Cholesterol 0 mg	0%
Sodium 55 mg	2%
Potassium 360 mg	10%
Total carbohydrate 40 g	13%
Dietary fiber 4 g	18%
Sugars 17 g	
Protein 4 g	

Vitamin A 130%	•	Vitamin C 15%
Calcium 6%	•	Iron 10%
Vitamin K 25%	•	Niacin 10%
Folate 6%	•	Magnesium 10%

• Percent daily values are based on a 2,000 calorie diet. Your daily values may be higher or lower depending on your calorie needs:

	Calories:	2,000	2,500
Total fat	Less than	65 g	80 g
Saturated fat	Less than	20 g	25 g
Cholesterol	Less than	300 mg	300 mg
Sodium	Less than	2,400 mg	2,400 mg
Potassium	Less than	3,500 mg	3,500 mg
Total carbohydrate		300 g	375 g
Dietary fiber		25 g	30 g

Calories per gram:
 Fat 9 • Carbohydrate 4 • Protein 4

Contains: Nuts, soy, wheat

The next two questions are based on this chart.

17. In addition to fiber, what type of carbohydrate is found in this product?

A) Fat
B) Potassium
C) Sugar
D) Folate

GO ON TO THE NEXT PAGE

18. Why might pregnant women wish to avoid this product?

    A) Pregnant women need more calcium than this provides.
    B) Excess vitamin A may prove toxic to pregnant women.
    C) Most pregnant women consume more than 2,000 calories daily.
    D) Pregnant women must not eat over 85 grams per sitting.

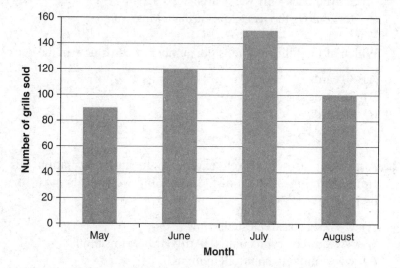

The next two questions are based on this graph.

19. In which month were the fewest grills sold?

    A) May
    B) June
    C) July
    D) August

20. How many more grills were sold in August than in May?

    A) 10
    B) 20
    C) 40
    D) 60

GO ON TO THE NEXT PAGE

21. Read and follow the directions below.

   1. Imagine a deck of 52 cards, ranging from twos through the face cards to aces, all in four equal suits—hearts, diamonds, clubs, and spades.

   2. Remove all of the red suit cards.

   3. Add back only the hearts.

   4. Remove the jacks, queens, and kings.

Which of the following tells the number of cards now in the deck?

A) 30 cards

B) 35 cards

C) 40 cards

D) 45 cards

22. A traveler uses a search engine to locate information on New Hampshire inns. Which of the following websites is most likely to be helpful?

A) www.seacoastrealestate.com/

B) www.directorynh.com/NHArt/NHMuseums.html

C) www.nhliving.com/lodging/inns/

D) www.newenglandinnsandresorts.com/

23.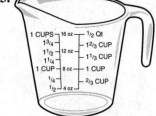

Based on the measuring cup above, which measurement is equivalent to $1\frac{1}{2}$ cups?

A) 8 ounces

B) 12 ounces

C) $\frac{1}{4}$ quart

D) 16 ounces

GO ON TO THE NEXT PAGE

The following form was sent to employees of a high-tech firm.

Professional Development Calculator

Name _____ Position _____ Department _____

Hours of Professional Development (30 required)

___ reading journals (list names) _____

___ coursework (list course/college) _____

___ workshops (list title/location) _____

___ virtual training (list title/site) _____

___ other (explain) _____

The next two questions are based on this form.

24. What is the purpose of this form?

    A) To suggest ways in which to improve job skills
    B) To name a variety of professional training sites
    C) To compare off-site and on-site training opportunities
    D) To record hours of training and advanced study

25. Based on the context of this form, what does *virtual* mean?

    A) Worthy
    B) Essential
    C) On line
    D) Edible

26. Blood-brain barrier, 234
    Blood groups, 155–158
    Blood plasma, 152–154
    Blood platelets. *See* Thrombocytes
    Blood pressure, control of, 130–134

    A student wants to learn more about type O blood. Based on this excerpt from a textbook's index, on which of the following pages should the student begin to look?

    A) 152
    B) 153
    C) 154
    D) 155

GO ON TO THE NEXT PAGE

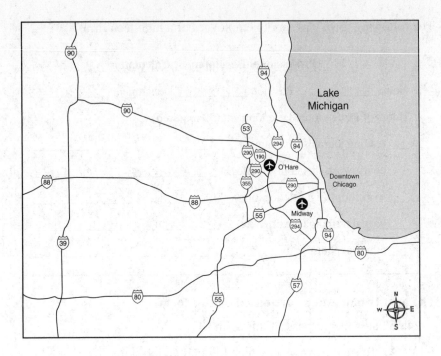

The next two questions are based on this map.

27. A traveler heading from downtown Chicago to O'Hare Airport might take which route?

A) Route 90
B) Routes 290 to 294
C) Routes 94 to 190
D) Routes 90 to 94

28. Midway Airport lies in which direction from downtown Chicago?

A) Southeast
B) Southwest
C) Northeast
D) Northwest

GO ON TO THE NEXT PAGE

29. Which of the following sentences shows the most logical sequence of events?

A) The scientist peered into the eyepiece for several moments, adjusted the focus, made a notation about what he saw, and placed the slide under the microscope.

B) The scientist made a notation about what he saw, placed the slide under the microscope, peered into the eyepiece for several moments, and adjusted the focus.

C) The scientist adjusted the focus, placed the slide under the microscope, made a notation about what he saw, and peered into the eyepiece for several moments.

D) The scientist placed the slide under the microscope, adjusted the focus, peered into the eyepiece for several moments, and made a notation about what he saw.

30. Chapter 3: Nations of Asia

    1. Southeast Asia
       A. Cambodia
       B. Vietnam
       C. Indonesia
       D. _____
       E. Malaysia

Examine the headings above. Based on what you see, which of the following is a reasonable heading to insert in the blank spot?

A) India
B) Japan
C) Afghanistan
D) Thailand

31. Begin with the word *trust*. Follow the directions to change the word.

    1. Change the first *t* to *c*.
    2. Change the last *t* to *h*.
    3. Change the *u* to *a*.
    4. Replace *cr* with *sl*.

Which of the following is the new word?

A) last
B) slat
C) crush
D) slash

GO ON TO THE NEXT PAGE

32. A resident of the city would like to express his opinion about an upcoming garbage strike. Which department of the newspaper should he contact?

A) Editorial
B) Business
C) Local news
D) Classified

33. Chapter 5: Hoofed Mammals

      A. Cattle and Relatives
      B. Horses and Relatives
      C. Elephants and Relatives
      D. Badgers and Relatives

Analyze the headings above. Which of the following headings is out of place?

A) Cattle and Relatives
B) Horses and Relatives
C) Elephants and Relatives
D) Badgers and Relatives

34. One of the research sources a scientist used for her paper was a primary source. Which one was it?

A) A review of the literature by a graduate student
B) A student's lab notebook from a nearby college
C) A recent article from *Scientific American*
D) An analysis of research in her field of study

35. A student writing a report wonders whether to use *that* or *which* in a particular sentence. Which of the following resources should the student consult?

A) *New Oxford American Dictionary*
B) *Webster's New World Thesaurus*
C) *The Art and Mastery of Punctuation*
D) *Fowler's Modern English Usage*

36. Her <u>altruistic</u> act aided many and cost her little but time.

Which of the following is the definition of the word *altruistic*?

A) Unusual
B) Selfless
C) Naive
D) Impending

GO ON TO THE NEXT PAGE

37. glow worms, 163
gnats, dark-winged fungus, 270, **271**
eye, 298
gall, 271, **271**
wood, 268, **269**

What is the purpose of using boldface on certain numerals in the index above?

A) To separate page references
B) To indicate the most important pages
C) To show a hierarchy of insects
D) To highlight pages with illustrations

38. Microcalcifications show up on mammograms as tiny, salt-like, white specks. They are not of particular concern unless they display certain patterns throughout the breast, in which case they may indicate a precancerous condition or even an early stage of breast cancer. In such a case, a doctor may call for a needle biopsy or stereotactic biopsy, and if those results indicate the presence of a low-grade tumor, a surgical biopsy may follow.

Based on this passage, when would a doctor call for a needle biopsy?

A) When microcalcifications first appear
B) When microcalcifications display certain patterns
C) When microcalcifications form a low-grade tumor
D) When a stereotactic biopsy indicates microcalcifications

39.

Based on the tape measure above, 4 centimeters is about equal to which of the following measurements?

A) 7.5 meters
B) 25 feet
C) $1\frac{9}{16}$ inches
D) 10 inches

GO ON TO THE NEXT PAGE

40.

Store	Location	Price per Pound
Wheeler's	5 miles away	$7
Fish Mart	10 miles away	$6
Chaney's	15 miles away	$5
Henley's	20 miles away	$4

Sara wants to purchase 20 one-pound lobsters for a party. If gas is $4/gallon, and she gets 20 miles to the gallon, which store should she visit to get the best all-around deal?

A) Wheeler's
B) Fish Mart
C) Chaney's
D) Henley's

SMOKE DETECTORS 281

SIGN LANGUAGE
See Translators & Interpreters

Di MARCO SIGNS
Specialists in illumination
and backlighting!
185 Elm St.

SIGNS
American Sign 15 Morton St 555-1284
Carbon Copies 87 Main St 555-2499
Di Marco Signs 185 Elm St 555-3434
Marshall Signs 24 Main St 555-3100

SKI INSTRUCTION
Bergen Skis Truxton Blvd . . . 555-3116
Donahue Trails 13 Pine Rd . . . 555-9495
SKIN CARE
Altima Spa 425 Morton St . . . 555-6880
Krystal's on Main 23 Main St . . . 555-8300
SMOKE DETECTORS
Alarm Service 280 Elm St . . . 555-2413

SIGNS—ERECTING & HANGING
American Sign 15 Morton St 555-1284

SIGNS—MAINTENANCE & REPAIR
Di Marco Signs 185 Elm St 555-3434
Marshall Signs 24 Main St 555-3100

KRYSTAL'S ON MAIN STREET
Full-service salon
nails, hair, makeup,
spa services
555-8300 Mon-Sat

SKATING RINKS & PARKS
Cass Park Rink 701 Judd Rd. 555-9411
JM Sports Complex College Pl. . . . .
www.jmcomplex.net 555-1414

The next two questions are based on this sample yellow page.

41. A customer wishes to receive a facial treatment after getting her hair cut. Which number should she probably call?

A) 555-6880
B) 555-8300
C) 555-1414
D) 555-3434

GO ON TO THE NEXT PAGE

42. Which two businesses are found on the same street?

A) American Sign and Carbon Copies
B) Marshall Signs and Cass Park Rink
C) Di Marco Signs and Alarm Service
D) Altima Spa and Donohue Trails

43.

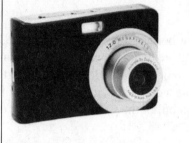

JOYPIX 180
12.0 megapixels,
self-timer, electronic viewfinder,
autofocus, tripod socket,
color LCD screen, brightness adjustment
$79.99

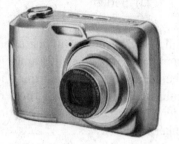

POWER SHOOT Z
14.0 megapixels,
date and time print, face detection,
autofocus, self-timer,
LCD screen
$84.99

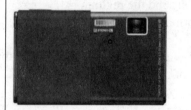

EASY SHOT WX
14.1 megapixels,
orientation sensor, auto scene selection,
face detection, self-timer, HD movie
recording
brightness adjustment, widescreen;
OLED display
$199.99

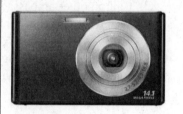

UPSHOT 920
14.1 megapixels,
electronic image stabilization,
self-timer, autofocus,
color LCD screen, easy-to-read menu
system
$149.99

A consumer wants a camera with face detection technology that is under $150. Which camera should he choose?

A) Joypix 180
B) Power Shoot Z
C) Easy Shot WX
D) Upshot 920

GO ON TO THE NEXT PAGE

44. After the party was over, we seemed to have a <u>surfeit</u> of seltzer and soft drinks remaining.

Which of the following is the definition of the word *surfeit*?

A) Facade
B) Excess
C) Upsurge
D) Series

Following a week of unrest along the border, the Secretary of State had an emergency meeting with ambassadors to Pakistan and Afghanistan today. She came away satisfied that the situation was under control and that the ambassadors expected no further violence as both sides joined in talks. The Secretary urged both ambassadors to monitor the situation and report directly to her.

The next two questions are based on this passage.

45. Based on the passage, which of the following is a logical prediction of what the Secretary of State will do next?

A) Join the peace talks between the two sides.
B) Express her displeasure in a press conference.
C) Call on other ambassadors around the region.
D) Wait to receive further information from the ambassadors.

46. Based on a prior knowledge of literature, the reader can infer that this passage was taken from which of the following?

A) A newspaper article
B) A folk tale
C) A persuasive essay
D) A history textbook

GO ON TO THE NEXT PAGE

47. A reader comes across an unfamiliar word in a textbook. Which of the following is the best place to find a definition?

A) The index
B) The appendix
C) The preface
D) The glossary

48. Read and follow the directions below.

1. Imagine three cups labeled A, B, and C.
2. Place a button in cup A.
3. Place two buttons in cup B.
4. Place three buttons in cup C.
5. Place one button from cup C into cup A.
6. Place half the buttons from cup A into cup B.
7. Place the buttons from cup C into cup A.

How many buttons remain in cup A?

A) Two
B) Three
C) Four
D) Five

GO ON TO THE NEXT PAGE

Hawaiian Water Tours

Departing daily from Honolulu on the southern coast of Oahu.

- Saturday—Fly to Kauai; sail and snorkel at Na Pali on the north coast

- Sunday—Fly to Maui; catch a ferry to Lanai or Molokai

- Weekdays—Catamaran tours of Oahu

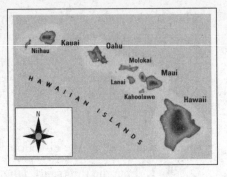

The next two questions are based on this advertisement and map.

49. Which of these islands is not available via Hawaiian Water Tours?

    A) Oahu
    B) Lanai
    C) Maui
    D) Hawaii

50. A vacationing tourist signs up for the Sunday tour to Lanai. In which directions will she travel?

    A) First southeast, then west
    B) First southwest, then slightly north
    C) Southwest only
    D) First northwest, then west

GO ON TO THE NEXT PAGE

Vaccinating Your Puppy

Every vet is different about the timing and order of vaccines, but all agree that you should not wait. By the time your pup is six weeks old, he or she should start the regimen of shots that are needed to stay healthy and sound into a ripe old age. Puppies receive some immunity from their mothers, but that drops off quickly, and they need commercially produced vaccinations to protect them.

Typically, the first vaccine is a combination meant to avoid a series of potentially fatal infections, including distemper, hepatitis, leptospirosis, parainfluenza, parvovirus, and coronavirus. The puppy may need booster shots at three- or four-week intervals.

At 12 to 16 weeks of age, puppies may be ready for a Lyme disease vaccine and a rabies shot. This latter shot is critical and required annually or biannually by law. Different states may require different timing, so be sure to check with your veterinarian.

The next three questions are based on this passage.

51. Which disease is *not* covered by the combination vaccine?

   A) Parvovirus
   B) Rabies
   C) Distemper
   D) Hepatitis

52. Based on the article, which shot would come last in the sequence?

   A) Distemper
   B) Leptospirosis
   C) Coronavirus
   D) Lyme disease

53. Why does the author recommend starting vaccines early?

   A) Smaller dogs need less medicine.
   B) Early vaccination is a state requirement.
   C) Puppies quickly lose their immunity to disease.
   D) Older dogs react poorly to some vaccines.

STOP. THIS IS THE END OF PART I.

Part II. Mathematics

36 items (32 scored), 54 minutes

1. $4\frac{1}{5} - 2\frac{2}{3}$

   Simplify the expression above. Which of the following is correct?

   A) $2\frac{1}{15}$

   B) $1\frac{4}{5}$

   C) $1\frac{2}{3}$

   D) $1\frac{8}{15}$

2.

Weekly Earnings	$560.40
Federal Income Tax	$64.63
State Income Tax	$27.67
FICA (Social Security, Medicaid)	$39.08

   The table above shows the deductions taken from José's paycheck.

   What is José's take-home pay each week?

   A) $691.78
   B) $495.72
   C) $468.10
   D) $429.02

GO ON TO THE NEXT PAGE

3.

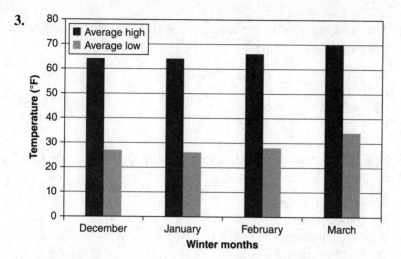

The graph above shows the average high and low winter temperatures in Nogales, Arizona.

The difference between high and low average temperatures is consistently

A) between 25 and 30 degrees.
B) between 30 and 35 degrees.
C) between 35 and 40 degrees.
D) between 40 and 45 degrees.

4. Find the total area of the figure shown.

A) 7.5 cm²
B) 12 cm²
C) 15 cm²
D) 24 cm²

3 cm   5 cm

5. $(3x + 2)(x - 2)$

Simplify the expression above. Which of the following is correct?

A) $3x^2 + 8x - 4$
B) $3x^2 - 2x - 4$
C) $3x^2 - 4x - 4$
D) $3x^2 - x$

6. In Downsville, a bus token cost 25¢ in 1990. This year, a bus token costs 75¢. What is the percent of increase in the cost of the token?

A) 50%
B) 75%
C) 200%
D) 300%

GO ON TO THE NEXT PAGE

7. A cake recipe calls for $2\frac{1}{2}$ cups of flour. How many cups are needed to make six cakes?

A) 12 cups
B) 13 cups
C) 14 cups
D) 15 cups

8. How many centimeters are there in 1 foot? (Note: 1 inch = 2.54 centimeters.)

A) 4.72 centimeters
B) 10 centimeters
C) 25.4 centimeters
D) 30.48 centimeters

9. What is the product of the numbers 0.25×0.4?

A) 0.01
B) 0.1
C) 1
D) 10

10. Takuo bought snacks from the vending machine. He paid $1.35 for cookies and got change from his $5. Then he paid another $1.75 for a bag of chips. How much money did he have left?

A) $1.50
B) $1.70
C) $1.90
D) $2.10

11. Leo spent these amounts on lunch each day this week: $4.50, $4.15, $4.85, $4.70, $5.05. What was his average daily expenditure for lunch?

A) $4.60
B) $4.65
C) $4.70
D) $4.85

12. Express $\frac{4}{5}$ as a percent.

A) 20%
B) 40%
C) 50%
D) 80%

GO ON TO THE NEXT PAGE

13. $\dfrac{2}{3} \times 2\dfrac{1}{8}$

Simplify the expression above. Which of the following is correct?

A) $1\dfrac{7}{24}$

B) $1\dfrac{5}{12}$

C) $1\dfrac{11}{12}$

D) $2\dfrac{1}{24}$

14.

Activity	Calories per Minute
Playing tennis	7.1
Walking at 3.75 mph	5.6
Running at 10 mph	15.0
Biking at 13 mph	11.2

This chart shows the calories burned per minute for each activity.

How many more calories are used in running for 20 minutes than in walking for 40 minutes?

A) 76
B) 66
C) 54
D) 24

GO ON TO THE NEXT PAGE

15.

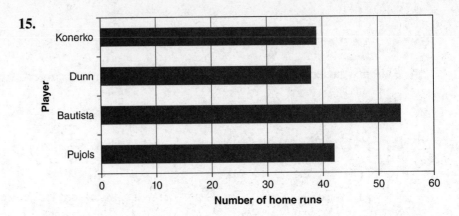

The graph above shows the number of home runs hit by the top league hitters in 2010.

Pujols and Dunn were the top National League hitters, and Bautista and Konerko were the top American League hitters. Which statement is true?

A) The top two American League hitters hit more home runs in all than the top two National League hitters.
B) The top two National League hitters hit more home runs in all than the top two American League hitters.
C) The top two American League hitters hit the same number of home runs in all as the top two National League hitters.
D) The top hitter in one league hit fewer home runs than the second best hitter in the other league.

16. How many liters are there in 500 milliliters?

A) 0.5 liters
B) 5 liters
C) 50 liters
D) 500,000 liters

17. Which answer is correct for the product of 0.22×0.75?

A) 0.00165
B) 0.0165
C) 0.165
D) 1.65

18. Four brothers have an average height of 70 inches. If three of the brothers each measure 69 inches, what is the height of the outlier brother?

A) 71 inches
B) 72 inches
C) 73 inches
D) 74 inches

GO ON TO THE NEXT PAGE

19. Which of these examples illustrates a negative correlation?

A) As a student's absences increase over the course of a year, his grades decline.

B) As more families move into the area, enrollment at the local school increases.

C) Older students tend to purchase cafeteria lunches more frequently than younger children do.

D) When enrollment in a local high school decreases, the number of faculty positions is cut.

20. Which type of graph would best compare the heights of two children over the course of a year?

A) Line graph
B) Histogram
C) Circle graph
D) Scatter plot

21. Order this list of numbers from least to greatest.

$$7,612; \ 7,162; \ 7,216; \ 7,621$$

A) 7,162; 7,216; 7,621; 7,612
B) 7,162; 7,216; 7,612, 7,621
C) 7,612; 7,621; 7,162; 7,216
D) 7,162; 7,612; 7,216; 7,621

22. Jenny's weight in pounds, w, is 20 pounds more than half that of her mother's weight, m.

Which of the following algebraic expressions best represents the statement above?

A) $\dfrac{w}{2} = m + 20$

B) $w + 20 = \dfrac{m}{2}$

C) $w = 2m + 20$

D) $w = \dfrac{m}{2} + 20$

23. $|x - 4| = 3$

Which of the following is the solution set for the equation above?

A) $\{1, 7\}$
B) $\{-1, -7\}$
C) $\{1, -7\}$
D) $\{-1, 7\}$

GO ON TO THE NEXT PAGE

24. A pharmacist is measuring individual doses of liquid medication for a prescription. Which would be an appropriate unit of measure?

A) Milliliter
B) Liter
C) Pint
D) Cup

25. A landscaping plan is drawn on a 1:50 scale. If a deck in the plan measures 12 cm by 10 cm, how large is the deck in real life?

A) 12 m by 10 m
B) 6 m by 5 m
C) 5 m by 2 m
D) 4 m by 3 m

26. Ninety-six percent of the class passed the exam with a C or better. If there are 50 students in the class, how many passed with a C or better?

A) 45
B) 46
C) 47
D) 48

27. At the concession stand, Joanie bought a hot dog for $1.25, popcorn for $1.35, and a drink for $2. She paid with a $5 bill. What is the least number of coins she could have received as correct change?

A) One
B) Two
C) Three
D) Four

28. Nurse Jackie checked a patient's temperature every hour for 5 hours, with these results: 102.2°F, 101.3°F, 98.9°F, 101.3°F, 101.5°F. What was the mode of this set of data?

A) 101.04°F
B) 101.3°F
C) 101.4°F
D) The data set has no mode.

GO ON TO THE NEXT PAGE

29.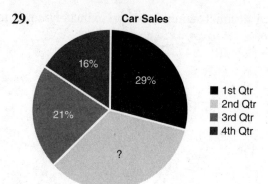

Car Sales

The circle graph above shows the percentage of car sales for one company across four quarters.

What percentage of sales took place in the second quarter?

A) 29%
B) 31%
C) 34%
D) 42%

30. $3\dfrac{3}{4} \div 1\dfrac{1}{2}$

Simplify the expression above. Which of the following is correct?

A) $2\dfrac{1}{4}$

B) $2\dfrac{1}{2}$

C) $3\dfrac{1}{8}$

D) $5\dfrac{5}{8}$

31. At the office supply store, Melissa bought a pen for $1.89, a notepad for $2.19, and two packs of pencils for $3.98 apiece. Which of the following is an accurate estimate of her expenditure at the office supply store?

A) $10
B) $12
C) $15
D) $18

GO ON TO THE NEXT PAGE

32. Which of the following decimal numbers is approximately equal to $\sqrt{90}$?

A) 8.9
B) 9.1
C) 9.5
D) 9.8

33. $x + 4 \geq 5$

Solve the inequality.

A) $x > 2$
B) $x \geq 2$
C) $x > 1$
D) $x \geq 1$

34. Of the students in Ms. Ludwig's ESL class, 25 are from China, 14 are from Ukraine, and 6 are from Mexico. What is the ratio of students from China to the total number of students in the class?

A) $\dfrac{2}{3}$

B) $\dfrac{2}{5}$

C) $\dfrac{4}{5}$

D) $\dfrac{5}{9}$

35. Cyrus has $26 in savings. His friend Lucas has $50. They want to pool their money to buy a new gaming device. If Cyrus puts in $8 each week from his allowance, and Lucas puts in $5 each week, which equation below shows how many weeks it will take for them to have an equal amount to spend on the device?

A) $26 + $50 = ($8 + $5)x$
B) $13x = $26 + 50
C) $8x + $26 = $5x + 50
D) ($8x + $5x) - ($50 + $26) = x$

GO ON TO THE NEXT PAGE

36. $15x - 12x + 8 = x + 24$

Which of the following shows the steps to use to solve for x?

A) $27x + 8 = x + 24$
   $23x + 8 = x$
   $22x = -8$

B) $3x - 32 = x$
   $2x = 32$

C) $3x + 8 = x + 24$
   $2x + 8 = 24$
   $2x = 16$

D) $15x - 12x + x + 8 = 24$
   $4x + 8 = 24$
   $4x = 16$

STOP. THIS IS THE END OF PART II.

Part III. Science

53 items (47 scored), 63 minutes

1. Which is the function of lysosomes?

   A) Respiration
   B) Digestion
   C) Movement
   D) Transport

2. Polydactylism, the presentation of extra digits on hands or feet, is carried on the dominant allele. In the case of two parents with polydactylism, what percentage of their offspring are predicted to manifest the anomaly?

   A) 25%
   B) 50%
   C) 75%
   D) 100%

3. Where might you find nonstriated muscle?

   A) Heart
   B) Tongue
   C) Bladder
   D) Thigh

4. The cheekbones are _____ to the nose.

   Which of the following correctly completes the sentence above?

   A) anterior
   B) proximal
   C) deep
   D) lateral

5. How does a transverse section divide the body?

   A) Into right and left regions
   B) Into upper and lower regions
   C) Into front and back regions
   D) Between the dorsal and ventral cavities

GO ON TO THE NEXT PAGE

6. The spleen is part of the _____ system.

Which of the following correctly completes the sentence above?

A) nervous
B) integumentary
C) lymphatic
D) urinary

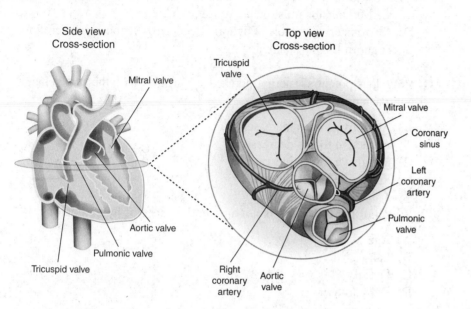

The next two questions are based on this diagram.

7. In the diagram, the pulmonary valve and aortic valves are open, allowing blood to flow

A) between the two ventricles of the heart.
B) from atrium to ventricle within the heart.
C) between the heart and the rest of the body.
D) between the atria in the heart.

8. Stenosis, or narrowing of a heart valve, may result in

A) abdominal pain.
B) blood clots.
C) edema (swelling) in organs.
D) irregular heartbeat.

9. Why are boats more buoyant in salt water than in fresh water?

A) Salt decreases the mass of the boats.
B) Salt increases the volume of the water.
C) Salt affects the density of the boats.
D) Salt increases the density of the water.

GO ON TO THE NEXT PAGE

---

10. Which is an example of inductive reasoning?

A) I heard the rooster crow at 5 A.M. this morning. I heard it crow at 5 A.M. every day this week. Therefore, roosters must regularly crow at 5 A.M.

B) Roosters have the ability to crow. My pet is a rooster. Therefore, my pet must crow.

C) Most farms have roosters. The McDonalds own a farm. Therefore, the McDonalds must own a rooster.

D) All roosters are male. Foghorn Leghorn is a rooster. Therefore, Foghorn Leghorn is male.

11. Why does potential energy increase as particles with the same charge approach each other?

A) Attractive forces increase.

B) Attractive forces decrease.

C) Repulsive forces increase.

D) Repulsive forces decrease.

12. Which of the following is *not* a potential cause of hypertension?

A) Age

B) Salt

C) Obesity

D) Dehydration

13.

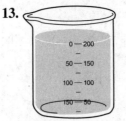

Which reading error would be expected and acceptable when using this beaker?

A) ±1 ml

B) ±2.5 ml

C) ±5 ml

D) ±25 ml

GO ON TO THE NEXT PAGE

14. Patient A, who weighs 150 pounds, steps onto a scale 20 times. The scale consistently weighs patient A as 165 pounds. What is true of the measurement?

A) It is valid but not reliable.
B) It is reliable but not valid.
C) It is both valid and reliable.
D) It is neither reliable nor valid.

15. Where are the acids known as gastric juices manufactured?

A) In the duodenum
B) In the stomach
C) In the pancreas
D) In the small intestine

16. What two body parts are connected by the esophagus?

A) Jaw and diaphragm
B) Stomach and trachea
C) Bronchus and larynx
D) Pharynx and stomach

17. During which part of an experiment might a scientist use a spectrophotometer?

A) Hypothesis
B) Analysis
C) Experimentation
D) Problem identification

GO ON TO THE NEXT PAGE

18.

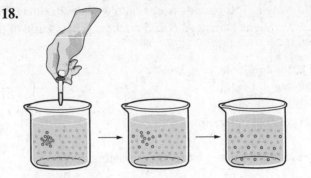

What does this diagram show?

A) Diffusion
B) Glycolysis
C) Homeostasis
D) Oxidation

19. How might vitamin D deficiency present?

A) As bleeding gums
B) As swollen extremities
C) As red patches
D) As crooked bones

20. Why is a "super-energy" diet that is high in fat but disallows carbohydrates likely to be ineffective?

A) Excessive fat may block the absorption of minerals.
B) Calorie counting is the only effective means of losing weight.
C) Protein calories are not as important as carbohydrate calories.
D) Carbohydrates are required to oxidize fat completely.

21. The specific heat of water is 1.0 calorie/g°C, and the specific heat of copper is 0.092 calorie/g°C. Which statement is true?

A) It takes more energy to heat water than to heat copper.
B) Water is a better conductor of heat than copper is.
C) A gram of water has greater density than a gram of copper.
D) Applying force to water will decrease its specific heat.

22. While conducting an experiment, a student determines that the majority of plants in the experimental group grew faster than those in the control group. This observation corresponds to which of the following steps in the scientific method?

A) Formulating a hypothesis
B) Collecting data
C) Analyzing data
D) Drawing a conclusion

GO ON TO THE NEXT PAGE

23.

PERIODIC TABLE OF THE ELEMENTS

1 H																	2 He
3 Li	4 Be											5 B	6 C	7 N	8 O	9 F	10 Ne
11 Na	12 Mg											13 Al	14 Si	15 P	16 S	17 Ci	18 Ar
19 K	20 Ca	21 Sc	22 Ti	23 V	24 Cr	25 Mn	26 Fe	27 Co	28 Ni	29 Cu	30 Zn	31 Ga	32 Ge	33 As	34 Se	35 Br	36 Kr
37 Rb	38 Sr	39 Y	40 Z	41 Nb	42 Mo	43 Tc	44 Ru	45 Rh	46 Pd	47 Ag	48 Cd	49 In	50 Sn	51 Sb	52 Te	53 I	54 Xe
55 Cs	56 Ba	see below	72 Hf	73 Ta	74 W	75 Re	76 Os	77 It	78 Pt	79 Au	80 Hg	81 Ti	82 Pb	83 Bi	84 Po	85 At	86 Rn
87 Fr	88 Ra	see below	104 Rf	105 Db	106 Sg	107 Bh	108 Hs	109 Mt	110 Ds	111 Rg	112 Uub	113 Uut	114 Uuq	115 Uup	116 Uuh	117 Uus	118 Uuo

■ = Alkali Metals   ▓ = Halogens   ░ = Noble Gases

RARE EARTH ELEMENTS

Lanthanides	57 La	58 Ce	59 Pr	60 Nd	61 Pm	62 Sm	63 Eu	64 Gd	65 Tb	66 Dy	67 Ho	68 Er	69 Tm	70 Yb	71 Lu
Actinides	89 Ac	90 Th	91 Pa	92 U	93 Np	94 Pu	95 Am	96 Cm	97 Bk	98 Cf	99 Es	100 Fm	101 Md	102 No	103 Lr

Which of these elements has the greatest atomic mass?

A) Au
B) Ba
C) I
D) W

24. Which of the following is an example of a nonsteroid hormone?

A) Cortisol
B) Estrogen
C) Epinephrine
D) Testosterone

GO ON TO THE NEXT PAGE

25. Who might be expected to demonstrate a rooting reflex?

    A) A patient with diabetes
    B) An infant
    C) A person with paralysis
    D) An adolescent

26. Which of the following muscles helps extend the elbow?

    A) Pronator terus
    B) Triceps brachii
    C) Extensor carpi radialis
    D) Brachialis

27. How does the endocrine system work with the reproductive system?

    A) The reproductive system transforms minerals into useful nutrients.
    B) The endocrine system determines the sex of the embryo.
    C) The reproductive system controls the growth of secondary sex organs.
    D) The endocrine system produces chemicals that regulate sexual function.

28. In an experiment conducted to compare the growth of three varieties of seed corn, the height of the corn is which type of variable?

    A) Dependent
    B) Independent
    C) Controlled
    D) Random

29. The organ system primarily responsible for regulating electrolytes is the _____ system.

Which of the following correctly completes the sentence above?

    A) endocrine
    B) urinary
    C) lymphatic
    D) reproductive

GO ON TO THE NEXT PAGE

30. Which of the following bones is part of the appendicular skeleton?

A) Sternum
B) Skull
C) Tibia
D) Hyoid

31. A bowler bowls a 5.5-kg bowling ball at 4.5 m/s. What is the ball's momentum?

A) $10 \text{ kg} \cdot \text{m/s}$
B) 16.2 km/h
C) $24.75 \text{ kg} \cdot \text{m/s}$
D) There is not enough information to calculate momentum.

32. Object A has a mass of 10 kilograms on Earth. If object A is moved to the moon, which is true about the mass of object A?

A) It does not change.
B) It increases.
C) It decreases.
D) There is not enough information to determine the answer.

33. Where does blood flow once it leaves the right ventricle?

A) Through the pulmonary artery
B) Into the right atrium
C) Into the left ventricle
D) Through the aorta

34. A student working in a laboratory graphed a correlation that indicated that a particular cancer cell's growth rate decreased over time, growing rapidly at first and slowing over a period of weeks and months. How would you describe this correlation?

A) Direct
B) Inverse
C) No correlation
D) Logarithmic

35. Which of the following would typically be used to treat thrombosis?

A) An inhalant
B) An analgesic
C) An antibiotic
D) An anticoagulant

GO ON TO THE NEXT PAGE

36.

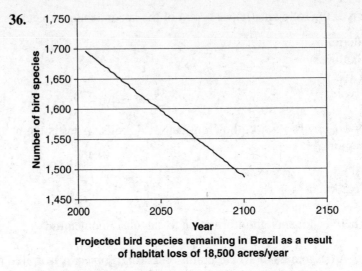

Projected bird species remaining in Brazil as a result of habitat loss of 18,500 acres/year

If habitat loss ceased altogether in 2050, what change might you see in the graph?

A) The downward slope might increase.
B) The slope might level off at around 1,600.
C) The graph would end at the year 2050.
D) The slope might angle upward again.

37.

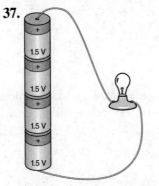

The diagram shows four 1.5-V batteries connected in series. What is the total voltage of the circuit?

A) 1.5 V
B) 3.0 V
C) 4.5 V
D) 6.0 V

GO ON TO THE NEXT PAGE

38. Which one is *not* a base?

  A) NaOH
  B) NH_4OH
  C) $Al(OH)_3$
  D) HCl

39. A boy jumps from a platform onto a trampoline. Once the boy hits the trampoline, what causes him to rise in the air again?

  A) Mass
  B) Inertia
  C) Gravitational force
  D) Reaction force

40. A ball hits the ground and bounces. As it rises back up, what does it do?

  A) Loses potential energy and gains kinetic energy
  B) Loses kinetic energy and gains potential energy
  C) Loses both potential and kinetic energy
  D) Gains both potential and kinetic energy

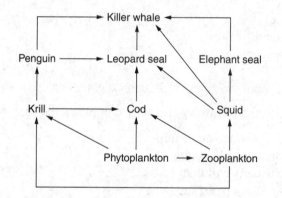

The next two questions are based on this diagram.

41. Which species represents the highest energy content?

  A) Killer whale
  B) Cod
  C) Phytoplankton
  D) Zooplankton

42. Overfishing of cod would be likely to have a rapid positive effect on which population?

  A) Krill
  B) Squid
  C) Leopard seal
  D) Elephant seal

GO ON TO THE NEXT PAGE

43. Most digestive enzymes belong to the class of enzymes known as _____.

Which of the following correctly completes the sentence above?

A) oxidoreductases
B) hydrolases
C) transferases
D) isomerases

44. The organ system primarily responsible for generating antibodies is the _____ system.

Which of the following correctly completes the sentence above?

A) endocrine
B) digestive
C) lymphatic
D) nervous

45. Where would you be likely to find the greatest concentration of Meissner's corpuscles?

A) Skull
B) Heart
C) Fingertips
D) Kneecaps

46. Unlike people with type 2 diabetes, people with type 1 diabetes _____.

Which of the following correctly completes the sentence above?

A) often produce no insulin
B) cannot absorb insulin
C) are usually children
D) may lack a pancreas

47. Which of the following structures is found in the inner ear?

A) Tympanic cavity
B) Eardrum
C) Auricle
D) Cochlea

48. What is the function of the nucleolus?

A) Transport
B) Ribosome production
C) Glucose production
D) Transfer of information

GO ON TO THE NEXT PAGE

49. Which are haploid cells?

   A) Gametes
   B) Blood cells
   C) Muscle cells
   D) Plant cells

50. The units of energy known as _____ are synthesized in the _____.

   Which of the following correctly completes the sentence above?

   A) ATPs; mitochondria
   B) ergs; cell wall
   C) ribosomes; DNA
   D) photons; stomata

51. Where might you find a fibrous joint?

   A) Skull
   B) Wrist
   C) Ankle
   D) Pelvis

52. What kind of tissue do the ganglia represent?

   A) Epithelial
   B) Connective
   C) Muscle
   D) Nervous

53. What is the function of a microphage?

   A) Stimulation of antigens
   B) Replication of red blood cells
   C) Production of perforins
   D) Digestion of pathogens

STOP. THIS IS THE END OF PART III.

Part IV. English and Language Usage

28 items (24 scored), 28 minutes

1. The steady breeze caused dry leaves to waft over the creek.

   What is the simple subject of this sentence?

   A) breeze
   B) leaves
   C) caused
   D) creek

2. Which sentence is written correctly?

   A) Maria has an unusual background, she started off as a student of geology.
   B) Maria has an unusual background; she started off as a student of geology.
   C) Maria has an unusual background she started off as a student of geology.
   D) Maria has an unusual background: she started off as a student of geology.

3. The word was unfamiliar. Bonita grabbed the dictionary. Bonita looked up the word. The word was in her textbook.

   To improve sentence fluency, how could you state the information above in a single sentence?

   A) When the word was unfamiliar, Bonita grabbed the dictionary and looked up the word in her textbook.
   B) Bonita looked up the unfamiliar word from her textbook, having grabbed the dictionary.
   C) Bonita looked up the word in the dictionary, which was unfamiliar in her textbook.
   D) Grabbing the dictionary, Bonita looked up the unfamiliar word from her textbook.

4. Which sentence from a medical report is most informal?

   A) Tests were conducted on March 10 and March 17.
   B) A prolapsed disk is compressing one or more nerves.
   C) Be sure to take your medication as suggested.
   D) The claimant should be restricted to sedentary work.

GO ON TO THE NEXT PAGE

5. Which of the following does *not* require citation in a published work?

    A) A well-known proverb
    B) A paraphrased restatement
    C) Data from another researcher
    D) Quotations from an author

6. Based on the root, something that is *polymorphic* has many ___.

Which of the following correctly completes the sentence above?

    A) colors
    B) parts
    C) lights
    D) shapes

7. The committee finished _____ report in time for the annual review.

Which of the following correctly completes the sentence above?

    A) its
    B) their
    C) it's
    D) they're

8. Do club members regularly ostracize people with working-class pedigrees?

What kind of sentence is this?

    A) Imperative
    B) Interrogative
    C) Exclamatory
    D) Declarative

9. Over the next few months, we _____.

Which of the following correctly completes the sentence above?

    A) listen and learn
    B) listening and learning
    C) had listened and learned
    D) will listen and learn

GO ON TO THE NEXT PAGE

10. I like the way the bride's stationery compliments her wedding décor.

What is the error in this sentence?

A) bride's
B) stationery
C) compliments
D) décor

11. The strident, overwrought monkeys made a raucous din as their unruffled keeper prepared their customary, nourishing repast.

Which words are redundant in the sentence above?

A) strident, overwrought
B) raucous, strident
C) customary, nourishing
D) din, repast

12. Which sentence is the clearest?

A) The car with the broken axle is now on blocks in his yard.
B) The car is now on blocks with the broken axle in his yard.
C) In his yard the car is now on blocks with the broken axle.
D) With the broken axle the car is now in his yard on blocks.

13. I noticed a number of workers from my car window who were repairing the road alongside the mall.

Which phrase or clause is misplaced in the sentence above?

A) of workers
B) from my car window
C) who were repairing the road
D) alongside the mall

14. In which of the following sentences does *deposit* mean "installment"?

A) Joe arranged for direct deposit of his biweekly paycheck.
B) The couple had saved enough to put a deposit down on the house.
C) After the storm, a deposit of salt crystals coated the glass door.
D) Miners chipped away at the rock, seeking a deposit of silver.

GO ON TO THE NEXT PAGE

15. The flock huddle against the wind that ruffles _____ feathers.

Which of the following correctly completes the sentence above?

A) its
B) their
C) it's
D) they're

16. Which of the following is an example of a correctly punctuated sentence?

A) We spent far too much time analyzing our choices and had little time left to act.
B) We spent far too much time analyzing our choices, and had little time left to act.
C) We spent far too much time analyzing our choices; and had little time left to act.
D) We spent far, too much time analyzing our choices, and had little time left to act.

17. Which of the following is the best definition of the word *megalith*?

A) Heavy volume
B) Large stone
C) Generous offering
D) Dangerous action

18. Which of the following is an example of a simple sentence?

A) Hardly anyone but Alice noticed the closetful of antique, embroidered dresses and robes.
B) No one else noticed, but Alice found the closetful of antique clothing.
C) While no one else was paying attention, Alice located an amazing closetful of lovely embroidered dresses.
D) The antique dresses and robes that Alice found were astonishingly lovely.

19. We found the movie clumsy, bland, and insipid; the actors, writers, and director seemed to be either fatigued or <u>contemptuous</u> of the audience.

Which of the following is the meaning of the underlined word above?

A) sympathetic
B) exhausted
C) scornful
D) insensitive

GO ON TO THE NEXT PAGE

---

20. Which of the following nouns is written in the correct plural form?

A) deers
B) syllaba
C) neuroses
D) waltzs

21. Which of the following is an example of third-person point of view?

A) Do you agree that the course is unexpectedly difficult?
B) Kyle and I finished the crossword puzzle in record time.
C) Most of us expect to work over spring break.
D) One should always follow the rules of the road.

22. That adorable baby is <u>always</u> so <u>angelic</u> at bedtime.

Which of the following correctly identifies the parts of speech in the underlined portions of the sentence above?

A) Adverb; adjective
B) Adjective; adverb
C) Adjective; adjective
D) Adverb; adverb

23. Which of the following sentences has correct subject-verb agreement?

A) All of our furniture was purchased in Tennessee.
B) Was any of his questions answered to his satisfaction?
C) Everyone in my nursing seminars seem well read.
D) Is both of the doctors available for consultation?

24. The play had been written by a committee of students.

Which of the following changes the sentence above so that it is written in the active rather than in the passive voice?

A) A committee of students had written the play.
B) The play was written by a committee of students.
C) The play had been written by students in a committee.
D) By a committee of students the play had been written.

25. Which of the following words is written correctly?

A) anti-depressant
B) ante-diluvian
C) un-appetizing
D) semi-invalid

GO ON TO THE NEXT PAGE

26. The teammates toss _____ caps in the air; _____ thrilled to have won the game.

    Which of the following sets of words should be used to fill in the blanks in the sentence above?

    A) their; there
    B) their; they're
    C) there; their
    D) they're; their

27. Nearly everyone in the class had completed the exam _____ but Peter felt that he ought to check his answers one last time.

    Which of the following punctuation marks correctly completes the sentence above?

    A) ;
    B) :
    C) -
    D) ,

28. <u>My friends and I</u> enjoy having the largest restaurant booth to _____.

    Which of the following options correctly completes the sentence? The antecedent of the pronoun to be added is underlined.

    A) us
    B) myself
    C) ourselves
    D) theirs

STOP. THIS IS THE END OF TEAS PRACTICE TEST 5.

TEAS Practice Test 5: Answer Key

PART I: READING

1. D	19. A	37. D
2. B	20. A	38. B
3. B	21. A	39. C
4. D	22. C	40. D
5. A	23. B	41. B
6. B	24. D	42. C
7. A	25. C	43. B
8. B	26. D	44. B
9. A	27. B	45. D
10. B	28. B	46. A
11. C	29. D	47. D
12. D	30. D	48. B
13. B	31. D	49. D
14. D	32. A	50. A
15. C	33. D	51. B
16. D	34. B	52. D
17. C	35. D	53. C
18. B	36. B	

PART II: MATHEMATICS

1. D	13. B	25. B
2. D	14. A	26. D
3. C	15. A	27. C
4. B	16. A	28. B
5. C	17. C	29. C
6. C	18. C	30. B
7. D	19. A	31. B
8. D	20. B	32. C
9. B	21. B	33. D
10. C	22. D	34. D
11. B	23. A	35. C
12. D	24. A	36. C

PART III: SCIENCE

1. B	19. D	37. D
2. C	20. D	38. D
3. C	21. A	39. D
4. D	22. C	40. B
5. B	23. A	41. C
6. C	24. C	42. A
7. C	25. B	43. B
8. D	26. B	44. C
9. D	27. D	45. C
10. A	28. A	46. A
11. C	29. B	47. D
12. D	30. C	48. B
13. B	31. C	49. A
14. B	32. A	50. A
15. B	33. A	51. A
16. D	34. B	52. D
17. C	35. D	53. D
18. A	36. B	

PART IV: ENGLISH AND LANGUAGE USAGE

1. A	11. B	21. D
2. B	12. A	22. A
3. D	13. B	23. A
4. C	14. B	24. A
5. A	15. B	25. D
6. D	16. A	26. B
7. A	17. B	27. D
8. B	18. A	28. C
9. D	19. C	
10. C	20. C	

TEAS Practice Test 5: Explanatory Answers

PART I: READING

1. (D) The sentence gives a reason for the main idea, so it is a supporting detail.

2. (B) The writer simply reports the story, which is so far unresolved. The best answer is choice B.

3. (B) The residents "have vowed to attend that meeting with charts and statistics in hand," indicating that Lister will face further opposition.

4. (D) Only choice D is something that cannot be proved or tested in some way. It is the speaker's belief, not a fact.

5. (A) The first paragraph states that he was "taken aback."

6. (B) Expository writing is designed to explain or inform.

7. (A) The topic sentence here introduces the entire passage by summarizing its content.

8. (B) The passage is primarily descriptive, although it also serves to invite readers to visit. It does not ask them to help preserve the site (choice C).

9. (A) According to the first paragraph, the victory "ensured America's sovereignty over the Louisiana Territory," implying that America's ownership was not a sure thing before that victory.

10. (B) The passage is primarily informative.

11. (C) Draw conclusions based on what is presented, not on guesses. The writer states, "Like all good historical restorations and most of our national historical parks, this one conjures up the history it celebrates," indicating that this is a desirable feature of historical sites.

12. (D) Space order moves the reader from place to place. The third paragraph does this by describing the panorama from left to right.

13. (B) The prefix *intra-* means "within" or "inside."

14. (D) Because the vaccine "contains no preservative or stabilizer," it must be used right away. The implication is that otherwise it may go bad or lose strength.

15. (C) The topic (choice A) is Lindy Barker, the main idea (choice B) is "Lindy Barker was memorable" or "some people linger in your memory," but the theme is memory.

16. (D) The paragraph seems to reflect upon something that happened to the writer and that event's meaning.

17. (C) Under "total carbohydrate," both fiber and sugar are named.

18. (B) Pregnant women should avoid excess vitamin A. Even if you did not know this, you should be able to answer the question through the process of elimination.

19. (A) The shortest bar is the one for May.

20. (A) The bar for August extends to around 100. The bar for May extends to around 90. $100 - 90 = 10$

21. (A) Start with 52 cards. Since the suits are equal in size, each one contains 13 cards. Removing all the red cards—diamonds and hearts—leaves you with 26 cards. Adding back the hearts gives you 39 cards. Removing the jacks, queens, and kings of hearts, spades, and clubs leaves you with 30 cards.

22. (C) Although choice D might help, choice C is specifically NH, or New Hampshire, and might be the better choice.

23. (B) Find the line for $1\frac{1}{2}$ cups and read across.

24. (D) The form is intended to be a record of professional development—training and coursework that improve one's job-related abilities.

25. (C) *Virtual* has more than one meaning, but the context here indicates that it refers to on-line training.

26. (D) Blood groups, of which type O is one, are discussed on pages 155 to 158.

27. (B) The easiest route would be to take 290 west and 294 north to the airport.

28. (B) Looking at the compass should tell you that Midway Airport lies to the south and the west of downtown.

29. (D) The logical sequence is to place the thing to be looked at under the microscope, adjust the focus so you can see it clearly, observe it, and take notes. Other sequences are possible, but only choice D is truly logical.

30. (D) Items A to E must all fit within the category of "Southeast Asia." On the list of choices, only Thailand (choice D) fits that category. India (choice A) is southern Asia, and Japan (choice B) is eastern Asia. Afghanistan (choice C) is considered part of south-central Asia.

31. (D) Working step by step: *trust, crust, crush, crash, slash.*

32. (A) In a newspaper, expressions of opinion belong on the editorial page.

33. (D) Badgers are not hoofed animals, so this heading does not fit.

34. (B) Original work and experimental results can be primary sources. The other choices are all secondary sources; they are one or more steps away from the original research.

35. (D) The question the student faces is which word to use in context. A dictionary (choice A) or thesaurus (choice B) is not designed to do this, and a book on punctuation (choice C) just deals with which punctuation mark to use. The student needs a book on usage (choice D).

36. (B) An altruistic act is one done unselfishly and without expectation of reward.

37. (D) Many books, particularly those that are field guides, as this one might be, use boldface type in the index to indicate pages that contain illustrations.

38. (B) When the spots first appear, they are not cause for alarm (choice A), but when they form patterns, a doctor may call for a needle biopsy.

39. (C) The top row of numbers indicates inches, and the bottom row indicates centimeters. Find the mark for 4 centimeters and read upward.

40. (D) If gas is $4 per gallon, and Sara gets 20 miles to the gallon, she can go 20 miles for $4. That means that the greatest distance she drives back and forth from a store will still only cost her $8 over the cost of the lobsters. Since the cheapest lobsters (at Henley's) cost $80 for 20, adding $8 to that is still less than the $100 for lobsters at the next cheapest store (Chaney's).

41. (B) Krystal's ad shows that it is a full-service salon, with hair treatments as well as skin care.

42. (C) Both of these businesses are listed on Elm Street.

43. (B) Three cameras (choices A, B, and D) are under $150. Of those three, only choice B has face detection technology.

44. (B) Only the word *excess* makes sense in context.

45. (D) Your prediction must be based on what is set forth in the passage. The Secretary of State "came away satisfied" and told the ambassadors to "to monitor the situation and report directly to her." It would be logical for her to wait to hear from them before doing anything more.

46. (A) The passage informs the reader about a current event.

47. (D) A glossary is a list of words and definitions in the back of an informational book.

48. (B) In problems of this kind, it may help to draw a picture. You start with three empty cups. After step 2, you have one button in cup A. After step 3, you have two buttons in cup B and one in cup A. After step 4, you have three buttons in cup C, two in cup B, and one in cup A. After step 5, you have two buttons in cup C, two in cup B, and two in cup A. After step 6, you have two buttons in cup C, three in cup B, and one in cup A. After step 7, you have no buttons in cup C, three in cup B, and three in cup A.

49. (D) Oahu (choice A) is the starting point for all tours. Lanai (choice B) is a potential part of the Sunday tour, and Maui is a required part of that tour. None of the tours go to the Big Island, or Hawaii.

50. (A) The tour starts at the southern coast of Oahu, flies southeast to Maui, and then goes by ferry west to Lanai.

51. (B) Rabies is a separate vaccine given later (at 12 to 16 weeks).

52. (D) Choices A, B, and C are mentioned as being part of the combination vaccine that is given first.

53. (C) The author makes this clear in the final sentence in paragraph 1.

Part II: Mathematics

1. (D) To subtract mixed numbers, first express them as improper fractions. In this case, $4\frac{1}{5}$ may be expressed as $\frac{21}{5}$, and $2\frac{2}{3}$ may be expressed as $\frac{8}{3}$. Next, find the common denominator—15. $\frac{21}{3} = \frac{63}{15}$, and $\frac{8}{3} = \frac{40}{15}$. Subtract the numerators: $63 - 40 = 23$. $\frac{23}{15} = 1\frac{8}{15}$.

2. (D) Subtract the deductions from the earnings to find the take-home pay. Deductions = \$64.63 + \$27.67 + \$39.08 = \$131.38. \$560.40 − \$131.38 = \$429.02.

3. (C) If it's consistently the same, you probably don't need to look at all four sets of bars. Pick an easy set: In March, the difference is about $70 - 35$, or 35. In February, the difference seems to be a bit greater, perhaps $66 - 28$, or 38. So the differences must be between 35 and 40 degrees.

4. (B) If the hypotenuse of the right triangle is 5 cm and the base is 3 cm, the height must be 4 cm, meaning that the area of the rectangle is 3 cm × 4 cm, or 12 cm^2.

5. (C) Start by multiplying the squares: $3x \times x = 3x^2$. Now multiply $3x \times -2$ and $x \times 2$, for $-6x + 2x$, or $-4x$ in all. Finally, multiply the final digits: -2×2, equaling -4. The solution is $3x^2 - 4x - 4$.

6. (C) First find the difference in price: 75¢ − 25¢ = 50¢. Then put the difference over the original price to find the percent change: $\frac{50¢}{25¢} = 2$, or 200%.

7. (D) Set this up as a proportion: $\frac{2.5}{1} = \frac{x}{6}$. You may cross-multiply to solve: $2.5 \times 6 = x$. $x = 15$.

8. (D) If 1 inch equals 2.54 centimeters, 12 inches (1 foot) equals 2.54×12, or 30.48 centimeters.

9. (B) Use common sense—0.25 is the same as $\frac{1}{4}$, so you are being asked to find $\frac{1}{4}$ of 0.4, which would be 0.1.

10. (C) Takuo started with \$5 and spent \$1.35 + \$1.75 in all. Subtract that total, \$3.10, from \$5 to get the amount left: \$1.90.

11. (B) To find the average, add the amounts and divide by the number of purchases: (\$4.50 + \$4.15 + \$4.85 + \$4.70 + \$5.05) ÷ 5 = \$23.25 ÷ 5 = \$4.65.

12. (D) Percents are fractions of 100, so you must multiply numerator and denominator by 20 to find the percent.

13. (B) Express $2\frac{1}{8}$ as an improper fraction: $\frac{17}{8}$. Then multiply numerators and denominators: $\frac{2}{3} \times \frac{17}{8} = \frac{34}{24}$. Finally, express this as a mixed number in lowest terms: $1\frac{10}{24} = 1\frac{5}{12}$.

14. (A) The calories burned in running for 20 minutes equal 15×20, or 300 calories. The calories burned in walking for 40 minutes equal 5.6×40, or 224 calories. The difference is $300 - 224$, or 76 calories.

15. (A) Arrange the data in a way that helps you compare. Pujols and Dunn were the top National League hitters, with approximately 42 and 38 home runs, or 80 in all. Bautista and Konerko were the top American League hitters, with approximately 54 and 39 home runs, or 93 in all. Statement A is true.

16. (A) One milliliter $= 0.001$ liters, so 500 milliliters $= 0.5$ liters.

17. (C) Multiplying two numbers with two digits to the right of the decimal point should result in a product with four digits to the right of the decimal point. However, in this case, the final digit, 0, is dropped off.

18. (C) Think of this problem as an equation, with the outlier brother's height represented by x: $(69 + 69 + 69 + x) \div 4 = 70$. You may solve by trial and error, or using algebra: $(207 + x) \div 4 = 70$, $(207 + x) = 70 \times 4$, $(207 + x) = 280$, $x = 280 - 207$, $x = 73$. Check by plugging 73 into the original equation: $(69 + 69 + 69 + 73) \div 4 = 70$, $280 \div 4 = 70$.

19. (A) A negative correlation is one in which the variables move in different directions, with one increasing as the other decreases. This is true only of choice A. Even choice D, in which both variables decrease, is a positive correlation, since both variables move in the same downward direction.

20. (B) A histogram, or bar graph, easily shows comparisons.

21. (B) $7{,}162 < 7{,}216 < 7{,}612 < 7{,}621$.

22. (D) Half Jenny's mother's weight equals $\frac{m}{2}$. Adding 20 to that leads to $\frac{m}{2} + 20$. For example, if Jenny's mother weighs 160 pounds, Jenny weighs $\left(\frac{60}{2}\right) + 20$, or 100 pounds.

23. (A) The bars mean "absolute value," which denotes the distance from zero on the number line and is always expressed as a positive number. $7 - 4 = 3$, so one of the numbers is 7. In addition, $1 - 4 = -3$, and the absolute value of -3 is 3, making the other number 1.

24. (A) Individual doses would be small, so a milliliter is a reasonable unit of measure.

25. (B) You can find the answer by setting up the easier of the two possible proportions: $\frac{1}{50} = \frac{10}{x}$, so $x = 500$ cm. Since 500 cm $= 5$ m, you should be able to rule out all of the choices but B.

26. (D) Solve by multiplying 50 by 96%, or 0.96: $50 \times 0.96 = 48$.

27. (C) First determine how much Joanie spent in all: $\$1.25 + \$1.35 + \$2 = \$4.60$. Subtract to find out how much change she was owed: $\$5.00 - \$4.60 = \$0.40$. There are many combinations of coins that add up to $\$0.40$; the smallest combination is 1 quarter $+$ 1 dime $+$ 1 nickel, for 3 coins in all.

28. (B) The mode is the most frequent number in the set.

29. (C) Add the other percentages and subtract from 100%: $29 + 16 + 21 = 66$. $100 - 66 = 34$.

30. (B) Express the mixed numbers as improper fractions: $\dfrac{15}{4} \div \dfrac{3}{2}$. Multiply $\dfrac{15}{4}$ by the reciprocal of $\dfrac{3}{2}$ to find the answer: $\dfrac{15}{4} \times \dfrac{2}{3} = \dfrac{30}{12}$. Express as a mixed number in lowest terms: $2\dfrac{1}{2}$.

31. (B) Rounding the numbers to the nearest dollar can help you estimate fairly accurately: $2 + $2 + $4 + $4 = 12. The best answer is choice B.

32. (C) You know that 9 squared is 81, and 10 squared is 100, so the square root of 90 must be right in between 9 and 10.

33. (D) You may solve this by trial and error, or you may work it out algebraically: $x + 4 \geq 5$, so $x \geq 1$.

34. (D) Add to find the total number of students: $25 + 14 + 6 = 45$. The number of Chinese students compared to the total is $\dfrac{25}{45}$. Expressed in lowest terms, that is $\dfrac{5}{9}$.

35. (C) The problem asks about a number of weeks, x, after which both boys will have an equal amount of money. Since Cyrus is starting with less but adding more each week than Lucas is, that day will eventually arrive. Only choice C demonstrates an algebraic solution: Cyrus's $8 per week plus his existing $26 will at some point equal Lucas's $5 per week and existing $50. If you were to solve, you would end up with $3x = 24, so $x = 8$ weeks.

36. (C) Do the easiest addition/subtraction first: $15x - 12x = 3x$. Subtracting x from both sides of the equation gives you $2x + 8$ on one side and 24 on the other. Subtracting 8 from each side gives you $2x = 16$, meaning that $x = 8$. Plug that back into the original equation to check:

$$15(8) - 12(8) + 8 = 8 + 24$$
$$120 - 96 + 8 = 32$$
$$24 + 8 = 32$$

Part III: Science

1. (B) Lysosomes are organelles in the cell that contain digestive enzymes. They help destroy damaged cells and digest bacteria and other biomolecules.

2. (C) If the trait is carried on the dominant allele, either an AA combination or an Aa combination results in the manifestation of the trait.

3. (C) Like skeletal muscle (choices B and D), cardiac muscle (choice A) is striated, or striped. The muscle in certain hollow organs (choice C) is smooth and not striated.

4. (D) The cheekbones are to the right and left of the nose, meaning that they are lateral to it, or away from the body's midline.

5. (B) A transverse section is a cross-section.

6. (C) The spleen uses lymphocytes and macrophages to filter out bacteria, dead tissue, and foreign matter.

7. (C) The two valves connect the heart to the pulmonary artery and the aorta, which carry blood from the heart to the rest of the body.

8. (D) Narrowing of the valves means that blood moves with difficulty out of the heart. Results may include chest pain, edema in the feet or ankles, and irregular heartbeat.

9. (D) Fresh water has a density of around 1,000 kg/m^3, whereas that of salt water is around 1,030 kg/m^3. The difference in density of the fluids makes objects in salt water more buoyant than those in fresh water.

10. (A) In deductive reasoning, a hypothesis follows from a set of premises. This is true in choices B, C, and D. In inductive reasoning (choice A), observations lead to a hypothesis.

11. (C) Unlike charges attract each other; like charges repel each other. As two like charges near each other, work is required to push them together, and potential energy increases.

12. (D) Hypertension, or high blood pressure, may be genetic, or it may simply progress with age (choice A). A high-salt diet (choice B) causes hypertension in some people, as do lack of exercise and excess weight (choice C). Dehydration (choice D) is more likely to cause hypotension, or low blood pressure.

13. (B) The smallest division of the measuring tool is 25 ml, so the expected error is $\frac{1}{10}$ of that.

14. (B) The measurement is reliable, because repeating it yields the same result. However, because it does not equal patient A's true weight, it is not valid.

15. (B) Gastric juices are manufactured in the cardia of the stomach. Gastric glands in the mucosa layer of the stomach secrete the juices, which are mostly composed of hydrochloric acid, potassium chloride, and sodium chloride.

16. (D) The esophagus lies behind the trachea and the heart and connects the throat (pharynx) to the stomach. It contains layers of muscle that push food along via peristaltic contractions.

17. (C) A spectrophotometer is a tool that measures light intensity. It would be most useful in the experimental phase, when data are being collected.

18. (A) Diffusion is the mixing or intermingling of molecules. Once the molecules are equally distributed, the solution is said to be in equilibrium.

19. (D) The disease known as rickets is a product of vitamin D deficiency and results in the softening and bending of bones.

20. (D) Omitting carbohydrates entirely makes fat harder to metabolize. Complete oxidation of fat requires oxaloacetic acid, a product of carbohydrate metabolism, so omitting carbohydrates entirely would make fat oxidation incomplete, allowing ketone bodies to accumulate in the blood.

21. (A) This is exactly the definition of specific heat, or heat capacity—a substance with a greater specific heat takes more energy to heat than one with the same mass but a lesser specific heat.

22. (C) Once the measurements have been made in the experimental phase, they may be compared and evaluated in the analysis phase.

23. (A) Gold (Au) has an atomic mass of 196.96655 amu. Barium (Ba) has an atomic mass of 137.327 amu. Iodine (I) has an atomic mass of 126.90447 amu. Tungsten (W) has an atomic mass of 183.84 amu.

24. (C) Steroid hormones are either corticosteroids, usually manufactured by the adrenal glands, or sex steroids, usually manufactured in the gonads. Nonsteroid hormones are usually amines or proteins—amino-acid-based rather than cholesterol-based.

25. (B) Infants use the rooting reflex, a turning of the face to the stimulus, to breastfeed.

26. (B) The triceps brachii on the back of the upper arm connects the humerus and scapula to the ulna and assists in extending the elbow. Of the other responses, choice A rotates the arm inward, choice C extends the wrist, and choice D flexes the elbow.

27. (D) The hormones produced by the endocrine system are critical in sexual development and reproduction.

28. (A) The dependent variable (choice A) is the one that is affected by the independent variable (choice B). In this case, the variety of the subjects is not affected by their growth, but their growth may be affected by the variety of the subjects.

29. (B) The body's electrolytes must be maintained at very precise concentrations. Excess water dilutes the body's electrolytes, whereas water restriction concentrates them. The kidneys regulate and help maintain the balance of water and electrolytes in the body.

30. (C) The appendicular skeleton is composed of the limbs, the pectoral girdle, and the pelvic girdle. Choices A, B, and D are part of the axial skeleton.

31. (C) Multiply velocity by mass to find momentum. $4.5 \text{ m/s} \times 5.5 \text{ kg} = 24.75 \text{ kg} \cdot \text{m/s}$.

32. (A) Mass is a property of an object and does not change. An object has the same mass on Earth as on the moon. Weight is a force based on gravity's effect on mass. On the moon, the weight of object A would be less than on Earth because of the reduced gravitational force.

33. (A) On the right side of the heart, blood enters through the vena cava into the right atrium, to the right ventricle, and then through the pulmonic valve into the pulmonary artery and to the lungs to be oxygenated.

34. (B) The rate starts high and decreases over time. As time increases, the rate decreases, making the correlation inverse.

35. (D) Thrombosis occurs when a blood clot blocks the flow of blood through a blood vessel. Anticoagulants are designed to prevent blood from clotting.

36. (B) The loss of species is connected to loss of habitat, so some kind of leveling off might be expected if habitat loss ceased.

37. (D) Attaching batteries in a series gives you a voltage equivalent to the combined voltage of all the batteries.

38. (D) Hydrochloric acid is a binary acid. Strong bases are frequently hydroxides, meaning that they contain covalently bonded oxygen and hydrogen. The presence of the hydroxide ion, OH^-, is often a clue that a compound is basic.

39. (D) Newton's third law of motion states that for every action, there is an equal (in size) and opposite (in direction) reaction.

40. (B) As the ball bounces back up, it loses velocity in kinetic energy and gains potential energy. No energy is lost; the total energy is equal to kinetic energy + potential energy.

41. (C) The highest energy content is in the producer level: in this case, phytoplankton.

42. (A) Cod eat krill, so reducing cod would most likely increase the amount of krill.

43. (B) Nearly all digestive enzymes work by adding a water molecule to break a chemical bond, making them hydrolases.

44. (C) Antibodies are formed when an antigen stimulates B cells, special lymphocytes, to produce specialized proteins that combat foreign substances or organisms.

45. (C) Meissner's corpuscles are mechanoreceptors that are sensitive to light touch and vibrations. They are widely distributed throughout the layers of the skin but are densely packed in the fingertips.

46. (A) In type 1 diabetes, which often starts in childhood but continues throughout life, the immune system destroys the cells that release insulin, causing insulin production to cease. In type 2 diabetes, the body loses the ability to absorb and use insulin. Insulin production may then decline steadily, causing insulin deficiency.

47. (D) The cochlea is a bony spiral in the inner ear. It transforms sound into signals that are transmitted to the brain. Of the other responses, choices A and C are found in the middle ear, and choice B is part of the outer ear.

48. (B) The nucleolus's main job is to produce ribosomal RNA.

49. (A) The haploid cells—cells containing a single set of chromosomes—produced via meiosis are the gametes, or sex cells.

50. (A) ATP (adenosine triphosphate), the main source of energy for cellular reactions, is generated in the organelles known as mitochondria.

51. (A) In a fibrous joint, bony elements are connected by continuous fibrous tissue, making the joint essentially immobile. In the skull, such joints are known as sutures. They are flexible in infants but become more rigid over time.

52. (D) A ganglion is a group of nerve cells, and therefore nervous tissue.

53. (D) A microphage is a small phagocyte that commonly consumes pathogens such as bacteria.

Part IV: English and Language Usage

1. (A) The subject is *breeze*, and the predicate is *caused*. The infinitive phrase *to waft* is a verb, but it represents what the breeze caused.

2. (B) The sentence is composed of two independent clauses. They could be written as two separate sentences, or they may be separated by a semicolon.

3. (D) Reading the choices aloud may help you determine which choice has a logical order of phrases and clauses. The least convoluted sentence is choice D.

4. (C) Any sentence written in the second person (addressed to "you") is considered to be informal.

5. (A) Proverbs, which have no obvious origin and are in common use, require no citation.

6. (D) The root *morph* means "shape," as in *morpheme* or *zoomorph*.

7. (A) The committee is working as a unit to produce a single report, so *its*, meaning "belonging to it," is an appropriate pronoun. If the committee worked as separate individuals to prepare a variety of reports, the pronoun might be *their* (choice B).

8. (B) An interrogative sentence asks a question.

9. (D) The next few months are in the future, so the appropriate verbs will be in the future tense.

10. (C) The bride's stationery does not compliment, or praise, her décor—it complements, or matches it.

11. (B) S*trident* and *raucous* both mean "loud."

12. (A) What is now on blocks? The car with the broken axle is now on blocks. Choice A makes the description and action clearest.

13. (B) Of all the choices, only choice B, if moved to the beginning of the sentence, would make the action clear: "From my car window, I noticed a number of workers who were repairing the road alongside the mall."

14. (B) When used as a noun, *deposit* has several meanings; among them are "money placed into an account" (choice A), "a layer of accumulated material" (choice C), and "a lode or vein" (choice D). In choice B, the word is used to mean "an installment toward a major purchase."

15. (B) The flock does not have feathers; the individuals in the flock have feathers. Since the flock is being treated as a group of individuals (as the verb *huddle* suggests), the pronoun should be plural.

16. (A) This is a simple sentence with a compound predicate. It requires no commas to separate its parts.

17. (B) The root *mega* means "large," and the root *lith,* as in *lithograph* or *monolith,* means "stone."

18. (A) A simple sentence has just one subject and verb. When in doubt, use the process of elimination. Sentences C and D contain dependent clauses, making them complex, and sentence B contains two independent clauses, making it compound. Only sentence A is simple.

19. (C) The base word in *contemptuous* is *contempt,* meaning "scorn."

20. (C) One *neurosis,* two *neuroses.* The other plurals should be *deer, syllabi,* and *waltzes.*

21. (D) Use the process of elimination if you are unsure here. Choices B and C are in the first person, and choice A is in the second person. *One* is an acceptable third-person pronoun.

22. (A) *Angelic* modifies *baby,* which is a noun. *Always* tells how often the baby is *angelic,* which is an adjective. Adverbs may modify adjectives.

23. (A) *All* (A) may be singular or plural, but in this case, it refers to *furniture,* which is singular. *Any* (choice B) may be singular or plural, but here it refers to *questions,* which is plural. *Everyone* (choice C) is always singular, and *both* (choice D) is always plural.

24. (A) Active voice expresses an action performed by a subject rather than an action performed on a subject. Here's a clue: If the person or thing doing the action is expressed within a prepositional phrase ("by a committee of students"), the sentence is likely to be passive. If the verb contains a form of *be* and the past participle of the main verb ("was written"), the sentence is likely to be passive.

25. (D) Choices A through C are closed (one-word) compounds. In general, a hyphen should separate a prefix from a base word that starts with the same letter as the last letter in the prefix, as in choice D.

26. (B) *Their* means "belonging to them." *They're* means "they are." *There* means "in that place."

27. (D) The sentence is composed of two independent clauses separated by the word *but.* That means that it is a compound sentence and requires a comma to separate the clauses.

28. (C) *My friends and I* could be replaced by the pronoun *we,* which might make the correct answer easier to spot. Having something "to ourselves" is an idiomatic phrase meaning to have it exclusively.